"A powerful book—one that will open many eyes and create the basis for essential change."

Norman Cousins
Anatomy of an Illness and *The Healing Heart*

"An insightful and comprehensive analysis of the special reasons so many women get hooked on drugs and alcohol and the special problems so many women have in . . . undertaking recovery. Informative, compassionate in tone, and well-written to boot, it is sure to be of enormous help to both professionals in the substance abuse field and to women seeking greater self-understanding."

Mary Ellen Donovan
Women and Self-Esteem

"*Women and Drugs* presents an underreported part of the drug picture in the United States today. Its personal perspective rivets the reader."

Joseph Michelson, M.D., co-author of
Illustrated Handbook of Drug Abuse Diagnosis

D1218589

"Very well-researched and eye-opening documentation."
   Cathleen Brooks
   President, National Association for Children
      of Alcoholics
   The Secret Everyone Knows

"Well-written, poignant, and eminently readable examples
of the various forms of alcohol and other drug addiction in
women. I hope they help many more like them to recover."

   Lucy Barry Robe
   Co-Starring Famous Women and Alcohol

"A much-needed revelation about chemically dependent
women's suffering from remorse, shame, and guilt."

   Chaney Allen
   I'm Black and I'm Sober

Emanuel Peluso & Lucy Silvay Peluso

WOMEN &DRUGS
Getting Hooked, Getting Clean

CompCare®Publishers

2415 Annapolis Lane, Minneapolis, Minnesota 55441

Peluso, Emanuel.
    Women & drugs: getting hooked, getting clean / by Emanuel Peluso
and Lucy Silvay Peluso.

        p.   cm.
    Bibliography: p.
    Includes index.
    ISBN 0-89638-144-7 : $9.95
    1. Women—United States—Drug use—Case studies.   2. Drug
abuse—United States—Case studies.   3. Narcotic addicts—
Rehabilitation—United States.   I. Peluso, Lucy
Silvay.   II. Title.   III. Title: Women and drugs.
HV5824.W6P45 1988
362.2′93′088042—dc19   88-2895
                                CIP

Cover design by Lillian E. Svec

Inquiries, orders, and catalog requests should be addressed to
CompCare Publishers
2415 Annapolis Lane
Minneapolis, Minnesota 55441
Call toll free 800/328-3330
(Minnesota residents 559-4800)

6   5   4   3   2
93   92   91   90   89   88

To Alice and Antony di Gesù

*The dark past is the greatest possession you have—
the key to life and happiness for others.
With it you can avert death and misery for them.*

Alcoholics Anonymous

To protect the anonymity of the women who shared their stories with us, their names and other identifying details have been changed.

Contents

Acknowledgments

Many people made this book possible. First, those personal friends who lent us their unfailing support, help, and ideas: Eleanor Widmer, Ph.D., Daniel Escher, William M. Hoffman, and Cynthia Lingg.

Many people in the alcoholism/addiction recovery field helped us: Belle Muschinske, M.A.; Judith Saalinger, M.S.; Judy Mahana, M.S.W.; Thomas A. Wright; Stephanie S. Covington, Ph.D.; Colleen Campbell, M.A.; Louise Lecklitner, M.S.Ed.; Jeanne McAlister; Teri Tucker Fredericks; Susan C. Richards, L.C.S.W.; Kate Martin; Audrey Mill; Cody Barrett, M.D.; Frances Larry Brisbane, Ph.D.; Karen D. Wells, Ph.D.; Dana G. Finnegan, Ph.D., C.A.C.; Emily B. McNally, M.Ed., C.A.C.; Brenda L. Underhill, M.S., C.A.C.; and Lynne M. Gardner.

And lastly, our profound gratitude to all the recovering women addicts, most of whom had never met us before, for sharing the deepest and tenderest part of themselves: their life stories. They overcame shyness, fear, and uncertainties to "give back" some of what they felt they had been given—their recovery. In the course of the tapings we laughed and wept together, and every woman, without exception, expressed the feeling that the story sharing process had been profoundly healing. To them, our best wishes for their continued journey in recovery.

1
Drug Addiction
A Women's Issue

Our own story

In the fall of 1984 we began sharing our own story of chemical dependency with mixed groups of newly recovering drug addicts at hospital treatment centers. At each meeting we told how, in the course of twenty-two years of addiction and fourteen years of marriage, we had used and abused marijuana, hashish, alcohol, cocaine, LSD and assorted psychedelics, amphetamines, hypnotics, painkillers and tranquilizers. We told how we had used drugs to wake up, to go to sleep, to improve sex, to improve conversation, to lose weight, to understand the meaning of life, to escape from life, to keep going, to relax, to get to the supermarket and back. And we spoke of lives riddled with screaming fights that brought the police, of languishing talents, casual sex, an alienated family, broken friendships, insensitivity to our children, ravaged health, and suicide attempts. And, through it all, there was the insane denial that made us sure that drugs were holding together and enhancing our lives, that the only problems we faced were "out there" in other people, places and things. It was they, we were sure, not drugs, which caused the loneliness, isolation, confusion, despair, anger, and sorrow we seemed always to labor under.

We told how our self-delusion, our arrogance and our yearning were such that, during the period of greatest strife and turmoil, we actually answered the telephone by saying "Peace!" And we told how, seven years ago, we heard the term "chemically dependent" from an old friend who had just gotten off drugs and we realized that was exactly what we were, that we hadn't been without at least one chemical coursing through our systems every day for years on

2 Women & Drugs

end. Until then, we had never thought of ourselves as addicts, and it never occurred to us that drugs were ruining our lives. But if taking drugs every day wasn't addiction, what was? And if our lives weren't in shambles, what were they? That was a moment of truth. We saw that we needed help. We told how we reached out for it.

Since then, the support we received from other recovering substance abusers has enabled us to turn our lives around, make amends to those we harmed, restore our health and get back to meaningful work. We told how our family life has stabilized, how our children can wake up to parents who aren't too strung out to take care of them. We've enjoyed reunions with family and friends. We've also made new friends and we feel comfortable around people, something we never felt on drugs. And we told how depression, anger and self-pity are no longer staples of our lives. Peace is no longer merely a word for us. It's a feeling, a place inside us where we can go. Of course, life has its ups and downs, but today we have a way of dealing with the down side without being thrown into a panic. We live with a sense of hope for the future.

"What about women?"

After one such talk, in a private drug treatment program in San Diego, a female patient came up to us and commented, "Your story was really something. But what about being a woman?"

"What do you mean?" we asked.

"You know, like the special problems women have. It's hard to talk about things like that with all the men here."

"Just stay away from the first drug one day at a time," we cautioned her, "and don't worry about side issues. They'll take care of themselves."

"Thanks," she said, squeezing our hands. We drove back home and got involved in the activities of the day, but something about this encounter bothered us. In speaking to recovering substance abusers we always tried to be rigorously honest, but we realized we had not answered this addict's question, "What about being a woman?" It now struck us how important her question was, and it occurred to us that no one was answering it, and perhaps altogether too few of us even knew what it meant.

The myths

In searching for the answer to her question, we would eventually interview over a hundred recovering women drug abusers. When we started this project we had certain preconceptions that we barely recognized. We believed, for instance, that a drug addict was a drug addict and gender was irrelevant. We believed men and women became chemically dependent for the same reasons and they used drugs in the same ways.

What we learned, however, was that drug abuse in women differs in many important respects: why they take drugs, where they get them, and how drugs affect them. We learned that women's special needs and life experiences have barely been addressed and are little understood either by family, friends and employers, or by professionals in the medical, counseling and law enforcement fields.

Most of us get our information about drug abuse from the popular media, where it is usually presented as a problem that affects and concerns males.

In 1976, for example, the National Institute on Drug Abuse published a comprehensive report called *The Lifestyles of Nine American Cocaine Users*. All nine subjects were male. In December, 1985, *Harper's Magazine* ran a twelve-page forum entitled "What Is Our Drug Problem?" Of the nine experts who took part, not one was a woman. In October, 1986, *Life* ran a front page story, "I Was A Cocaine Addict. What Happens When Nice Guys Get Hooked." And during the 1984-1985 prime time TV season, men made up three-quarters of the hard liquor drinkers, and two-thirds of prescription drugs users.[1]

In the occasional story that shows a woman using drugs, she is routinely pictured as the exception in a man's domain, and her addiction is patly explained: she is the runaway girl who falls under the influence of depraved men; she is the streetwalker whose exploitation and lack of moral fiber lead to a heroin overdose; she is the glamorous star confessing in *People* magazine how the pressure of fame and wealth got her hooked on alcohol and tranquilizers.

For those of us who have gotten our information about drug abuse from more academic sources, the picture is surprisingly similar. Almost all studies of drug abuse among the general population have included a disproportionate number of men in their samples, either because of the questions they ask ("Do you use drugs to enhance your sexual potency?") or their settings, where men are in the majority, such as county jails.

If in fact there *were* too few women drug abusers to warrant separate study, such one-sidedness might make sense. But, as recovering drug abusers ourselves, we have met literally scores of women, neither starlets nor harlots, who had been chemically dependent. These ordinary women—housewives, teachers, business-women—are generally not part of the public's conception of drug abusers. Yet, statistics assembled by federal agencies, particularly the National Institute on Drug Abuse (NIDA), a kind of clearinghouse for the latest information on drug abuse, clearly contradict the popularly held belief that addiction is a man's territory. In fact these statistics and others draw an alarming picture of the scope of drug abuse among women:

- A national survey of high school seniors showed that nonmedical use of stimulants is greater among the female students.[2]

- In 1984, forty-two percent of the callers to the 800-COCAINE helpline were *women,* an increase of eighteen percent over 1983.

- Women spend twice as much money per week on cocaine as men do.[3]

- Nationally, heroin addiction has increased at a faster rate for *women* than for men.[4]

- Twice as many *women* as men wind up in hospital emergency rooms due to drug overdoses.[5]

- Half of all drug-related suicides occur among *women,* most of whom are over thirty-five.[6]

- Alcoholic women outnumber alcoholic men in both completed and attempted suicides.[7]

- One out of every three new members of AA is a woman.[8]

- Women represent half of all alcohol drinkers and fifty-five percent of all wine drinkers. In 1984 they spent twenty billion dollars on alcoholic beverages.[9]

- Eighty of every ten thousand children born in New York City are born drug addicted because of their mothers' drug abuse, six times the rate of the midsixties.[10]

- Drug and alcohol abuse have pushed up the female arrest rates in California by more than thirty-three percent since the mid-seventies.[11]

- Finally, for the first time in our history, the rate at which new cases of addiction are being identified is greater among *women*.[12]

What this book is about

In view of the alarming scope of drug abuse among women, and the misplaced sense of hopelessness that often surrounds the subject, we felt that a book about ordinary women who had gone through and *recovered* from drug abuse was long overdue. We felt it should be a book that allowed chemically dependent women to tell their stories in their own words; one which would offer hope and inspiration to other women drug abusers, and at the same time bring some helpful insight to those who are watching a friend or loved one succumb to addiction.

For our purposes, we thought it best to deal with only those mood-altering substances that a vast majority of people would at present consider addictive drugs. We left out such potent substances as caffeine and nicotine because there is generally less social censure attached to their abuse. All the drugs which we decided to include, then, are either presently illegal or controlled: cocaine, barbiturates, Valium, marijuana, diet pills, speed, narcotic painkillers, heroin and civilization's oldest known drug, alcohol.

The drug of choice

We knew that most people who use drugs do not limit themselves to just one particular drug. We had read that fifty percent of people entering treatment centers today were poly- or cross-addicted. Forty percent of women in AA report being addicted to at least one other drug than alcohol. One woman told us, "There was an order in which I took drugs—the order in which they came on the market."

Nevertheless, regardless of how many chemicals a person played around with, and the variety could be literally staggering, one drug of choice usually came to the fore and became the most important substance in a chemically dependent woman's life. Each woman's story, therefore, centers around one particular drug of choice.

We assumed when we plunged into research for this book that there would be mountains of previous publications to guide us. We did find many volumes about alcoholism and a few chapters buried here and there in books about drugs in general that addressed some of the issues in female addiction. But after searching through medical libraries and stacks of feminist literature, we uncovered fewer than half a dozen reliable books devoted to women and the full range of addictive substances. It was as if an enormous catastrophe, involving millions of people, had failed to make the evening news. Was it simply an oversight?

Family denial

It was very clear, once we started interviewing women for this book, how such an "oversight" operated in the individual lives of our chemically dependent women. A Valium addict told how her parents refused to see that her suicide attempt had any relation to a drug problem: "In fact, my mother used to give me a lot of the pills. She also used Valium and she was quite willing to share her supply . . . My mother and dad felt that if I would straighten up and be Donna Reed, everything would be fine." The mother of our alcoholic was convinced that all her daughter needed to stay sober was "a few weeks' rest in a peaceful environment." The husband of our barbiturate addict was certain that as long as he doled out her daily ration of pills, "the situation was being beautifully controlled." When she finally took a crowbar to the family safe and took possession of her stash, he never again mentioned safe or stash.

Almost every woman we spoke to had a similar story about how parents, husband or children hid her drug abuse from the outside world, downplayed the seriousness of it, took it as a passing phase, or simply turned away from it.

If we multiply this dynamic millions of times within this country, the result is what one National Institute on Alcoholism and

Alcohol Abuse publication calls "a silent conspiracy of protection and denial."

We spent a lot of time wondering, what is a family's real stake in hiding a woman's drug problem? Obviously women were not being "protected." In fact, the very opposite is true. As treatment director Ruth Oakley wrote: "Men sometimes let their wives die rather than embarrass the family by bringing the problem into the open. It's the easy way out—and it happens."

A silent conspiracy

It was after reading what women themselves had written about chemical dependency that we understood the underlying reasons for a family's silence. In her book, *The Invisible Alcoholics,* Marian Sandmaier writes that, "When a woman is chronically drunk, she loses a large measure of the control that is absolutely necessary to the performance of her rigidly defined functions. And . . . there is no telling what taboo she will break next, what tacit agreement between the sexes she might expose and reject."[13]

Women are cast as the bearers of virtue in our society. We expect, even demand of them, a greater degree of morality and self-discipline in all areas of human endeavor. Their sexuality must be tempered with restraint, their ambition must be modified by diffidence, their intelligence must be sweetened by charm. When First Lady Betty Ford publicly admitted her addiction to drugs and alcohol, Sandmaier reports, some people angrily cancelled their subscriptions to those newspapers that carried the story. Such outrage betrays the emotional stake that parts of our society have in maintaining the image of a virtuous, self-disciplined womanhood. In the phrase of researcher Joan Curlee, "It is not easy to admit that the hand that rocks the cradle might be shaky." Drug counselor Judy Mahana told us, "For every woman drug addict hiding in a closet, there are usually several family members leaning against the door."

Women's drug abuse inevitably brings the problem of addiction out of the streets and bars and into the living room and nursery. In exploring its prevalence, in searching for its causes, we threaten to expose the dark underside of our archetype of contentment, the all-American Ozzie and Harriet family. "Women's addiction," a female therapist told us, "is a shameful reflection on the family members."

In interview after interview, we saw just how onerous, even deadly, society's projection of an angelic womanhood was. In failing to live up to this image, the chemically dependent women we spoke to all felt that they had failed miserably as human beings, that they had let down themselves and their families. "That's why women are more ashamed than men addicts," observed Ms. Mahana. "They feel more degraded. They feel they've lost their family's love and, because they can't stop taking drugs, their only alternative is to hide."

One woman told us, "I felt it was my fault . . . After all, I'm just the wife. I'm a woman who is supposed to make the beds and keep the house running, and he's the breadwinner. And basically how I felt is: 'and I'm the nothing.' Which led me to take more pills."

A Valium addict told us, "While I was under the influence, I'd start feeling really guilty and felt like I had been a bad mother and a bad wife . . . I always thought it was my problem, my fault. I did it. I was wrong and bad."

To avoid the censure of family, friends and society as a whole, women learn to hide their addictions. One alcoholic said, "You know, women hide it real well because we have to look good on the outside so no one will know how sick we are. That's one of the reasons it takes us so long to get to treatment because people don't see how sick we are. Because we look good. Women are trained to have their outsides look good anyway, so we just make sure we look *real* good."

The medical connection

Although prescription drugs are the focus of only four stories in this book, they played an important role in virtually every woman's story. Almost all our recovering women had been dependent on at least one of them, even if it was not their drug of choice. Cocaine abusers used tranquilizers to come down; alcoholics used Valium to get through the morning without a drink, or amphetamines to chase away morning hangovers.

Because legal drugs are just that—legal—they encourage a kind of warped thinking. A Valium addict put it this way: "If a doctor wrote it out, that meant it was innocent and harmless. And so I thought, if it was a prescription, somehow I just didn't connect it to be really drug taking, per se."

This is denial on a grand scale, and social attitudes reinforce it. In short, when a women is stoned out of her mind on doctor's orders, she's not an addict, she's a patient.

But the fact is that this legalized addiction is part and parcel of the silent conspiracy. We have in our midst millions of women whose dependence on prescription chemicals has been rendered invisible. They are hidden in plain sight.

Women are the primary consumers of medical care. They go to doctors' offices, for themselves and for their families, seven times as often as men do. And many women turn to their family doctors for more than physical problems. They bring to them emotional and lifestyle dilemmas. Since ninety-three percent of all physicians are male, most women are being treated for a broad range of women's issues by someone who has, at best, only a theoretical understanding of what these issues are. All the doctor really knows is that he is expected to come up with a solution. And, as one doctor put it, "It takes thirty seconds to write the prescription and thirty minutes not to."

Also, writing a prescription has become, in large measure, a necessary ritual. Many of us may feel shortchanged if a doctor doesn't give us one. A woman who goes to her doctor for depression, for instance, isn't asked, "What did he *do* for you?" She is asked, "What did he *give* you?"

One woman after another told us how, on leaving the doctor's office with prescription in hand, instant relief guaranteed, she stopped looking for the causes of her anxiety, pain, lethargy or unhappiness. She returned to her job or family where nothing had really changed, yet everything seemed different. She had been given the message that there was nothing wrong with her life situation or relationships, but rather there was something wrong with *her,* and her drug would now fix it. Her lifestyle problem had been transformed into a medical problem.

The abuses in treating women with prescription drugs is only beginning to reach public consciousness, but it is a practice whose roots reach back to the previous century. In 1894, one physician wrote, "We have an army of women in America dying from the opium habit—larger than our standing army. The [medical] profession is wholly responsible for the loose and indiscriminate use of the drug."[14]

In a classic study two doctors observed:

> ". . . the ease with which pain could be relieved through the hypodermic administration of the drug, the time it saved the physician in his busy rounds, the contentment it brought the patient, and above all, the all too common inclination to relieve symptoms rather than cause, contributed to increase the practice (of opium use) . . . by leaps and bounds wherever medicine was practiced.[15]

Today, only the drugs have changed. The issue is the same.

- Sedatives and diet pills have virtually become "women's drugs," with women taking seventy percent of the former and eighty percent of the latter.
- In 1978, thirty-six million women had taken legally prescribed tranquilizers, and twelve million had taken stimulants, outnumbering men two to one. An additional sixteen million had used sedatives.[16]
- *Two-thirds* of the more than two hundred million mood-altering drug prescriptions are written for women.[17]
- From two to four million women are addicted to legal drugs.[18]
- According to Dr. Robert S. Mendelsohn, Chairman of the Medical Licensing Committee for the State of Illinois, twelve million new women will be "lured into this medical merry-go-round" in an average year.[19]

Are these drugs serving any purpose? Are they solving any problems, curing any illnesses? One researcher answered this way:

The assumption that the "therapeutic" use of psychotropic drugs is beneficial is made so firmly that few have dared to question it . . . No proof exists to show that they provide any therapeutic benefit at all, unless a pleasurable effect is taken as synonymous with a therapeutic alleviation of distress. That the *feeling* of benefit cannot be assumed to be beneficial should be obvious . . . nevertheless this would seem to be the sole basis on which the psychotropics have been judged by patient and physician alike . . . the patient is more likely to be female than male.[20]

The prescribing of drugs to women has grown completely out of bounds. In 1982, a U.S. Food and Drug Administration survey found that participating physicians had written prescriptions for *every patient* they had seen the preceding week. Researchers have suggested that a doctor sometimes selects a drug because of his attitudes, not because of his patients' conditions or needs. We found cases where women were given downs on one visit to a doctor and ups on the next.

Expedience aside, why do doctors give so many women so many drugs? The answer may be simply that doctors' views toward women are reflective of society's attitudes as a whole; namely, a woman needs something to make her "normal":

- In 1975 the Task Force on Sex Bias and Sex Role Stereotyping in Psychotherapeutic Practice found that traits judged "normal" for the male are also judged "normal" for all people. Traits judged "feminine" are considered neither "normal" nor "ideal." [21]

- A 1977 survey of attitudes about problem drinkers and their spouses concluded that men and women were equally stigmatized for alcohol abuse, except in one critical area. Women alcoholics were rated *significantly more hopeless* than male alcoholics, even though statistics clearly belie that attitude.[22]

- In a survey of 161 physicians involved in alcoholism treatment, doctors generally characterized their chemically dependent women patients as more hostile, angry, unhappy, self-centered, withdrawn, depressed, more subject to mood swings, more emotional, lonely, nervous, more sensitive with less insight, *not as likable as men,* and limited by their biology![23]

- Given the same set of symptoms, women are twice as likely as men to be given a drug.[24]

It can hardly surprise us, then, that a profession laboring under this lopsided paradigm of womanhood—less likable, more sensitive, biologically cursed and hopeless to boot!—has resulted in what one counselor called "typical *Ms*treatment."

And for women trying to get off drugs, most doctors can offer little help. One doctor described how little he knew about drugs as the 4-2-1 rule: in *four* years of medical school he spent *two* hours on the nation's number *one* health problem.

New hope

While the picture we have formed of women's fate at the hands of medical practitioners may seem bleak, we've also seen that things are changing. Most of the women we spoke with are taking a less passive and obedient role. They are being encouraged to question a doctor's decision to use a psychotropic drug; some are seeking out doctors who are known to be less than trigger-happy with their Rx pads; they have begun to ask what alternatives there are to a recommended mode of treatment; they are demanding facts, not bland assurances, about the addictive potential and the side effects of prescribed drugs.

In fact, many of the attitudes that have perpetuated the silent conspiracy for the past hundred years—misunderstanding, isolation, and denial—are being overcome today by the brave efforts of women counselors, women researchers and, most of all, recovering women themselves.

This book has ten true-life stories, each story preceded by a profile on that woman's drug(s) of choice. These ten women have gone through the pain and anguish of drug dependency and have reclaimed their lives. In the midst of despair, each of them found the strength and hope to change. And each felt the greatest service she could render other women trapped in the cycle of drug abuse was to tell her story with fearless honesty. In doing so, these recovering women break through the deadly silence and neglect so many chemically dependent women presently suffer.

The stories that follow will introduce you to an extraordinarily diverse group of women. Some were raised in poverty; others were brought up in middle-class comfort; one spent her girlhood amid extravagant wealth. Some stopped their formal education at high school; others have attained Ph.D's. Each story has its own dramatic surprises.

The women in this book, by their courage and honesty, bring hope to us all.

2

Alcohol
Jill's Story

The Oldest Known Drug

American women's use of alcohol is escalating at an alarming rate. According to the National Institute on Alcoholism and Alcohol Abuse (NIAAA), women are drinking at an earlier age, drinking more than ever, and suffering from alcoholism in ever-increasing numbers.

Drinking among young women and teen-age girls is more common than among any other age group. Nearly three out of four high school girls drink, as do more than eight out of ten college women. As many as one-third of these young women may be problem drinkers.[1]

There are an estimated twelve million alcoholics in the United States, an increase of twelve percent since 1980.[2] Conservative estimates say that no more than one-fourth of all alcoholics are female. But cirrhosis of the liver, the only hard evidence of alcoholism, is found in women and men at a ratio of one to one.[3]

This same one-to-one ratio seems to be true in alcohol consumption. According to one liquor trade expert, half of all spirits and wine drinkers are women. In 1984, women spent twenty billion dollars on alcohol. By 1994, they will spend an estimated thirty billion dollars a year.[4]

Throughout Western history, women's use of alcohol has been surrounded by an aura of moral degradation and illictness. In ancient Rome, a woman could be stoned to death for drinking wine.[5] In nineteenth century America, alcohol was seen as "degrading the fairest and the loveliest of the creation to the level of the brutes," and destroying "every holy instinct and every womanly shame."[6,7]

Even today, popular culture teaches us that alcohol belongs to men. In TV ads and movies, in ballparks and barrooms, alcohol seems to make a man's life richer and imbues it with a golden glow of camaraderie. Men are free to glamorize its use as a sex-role enhancer, a social disinhibitor, and a seducer's tool. Women's use is expected to be moderate, discrete, sensible, and free from physical effect. In short, it must be ladylike.

This double standard binds the growing numbers of female alcoholics to a vicious cycle of denial. Whereas the public nature of a man's drunkenness may bring him up against authorities, kin, and peers, any of whom may confront him with his alcohol abuse, women are more often private drinkers. Typically, a woman feels a sense of shame about her "unladylike" behavior and, fairly early in her drinking, she tries to hide it. Even when she is ready to identify her drinking as problematic, family, friends and professional care-givers discourage her from admitting what is to them inadmissible.[8]

And so she is often treated for marital problems, depression, or financial difficulties. She is given tranquilizers, advice, or a pat on the back. The only thing she is not typically given is an equal opportunity for proper treatment. In 1984 there were more than 5,500 alcohol and drug treatment programs for men. There were fewer than four hundred for women.[9] And despite the rise of alcoholism among women, the male-female ratio of alcoholic diagnoses in mental health facilities remains at about five to one.[10]

This discrepancy is all the more poignant when we realize that alcohol seems to effect a woman's body and mind more quickly and more devastatingly than a man's. Even when women start to drink later in life than men, they show up at alcoholic treatment centers at approximately the same age. Their decline is telescoped. [11]

The reasons for this rapid decline are physical and psychological. Because a woman's body has a greater proportion of body fat and less body water, alcohol enters her system less diluted. Women get drunker, faster.[12] They also develop alcohol-related diseases— liver disorders, obesity, high blood pressure, malnutrition, memory loss, numbness of extremities and alcoholic hepatitis—faster, even though they drink half as much as men.[13] In one study, the mortality rate from cirrhosis among male alcoholics was eleven times that of the general population. Among women alcoholics, the rate was twenty-five times greater.[14] Alcoholic women under forty-five can have bone densities like those usually found in women of seventy.[15]

Alcohol has also been implicated in breast cancer, the second leading cause of death from malignancies among American women. Two long-term studies published in 1987 indicated that drinking even moderate amounts of alcohol increases a woman's chances of developing breast cancer by fifty percent, and taking more than eight drinks a week raises her chances by as much as 150 percent.[16,17] Other studies have found that women who drink heavily have a two hundred percent increased risk of breast cancer.[18]

Psychologically, women drinkers fare no better. They have lower self-esteem than comparable groups of alcoholic men. Most report diminished sexual interest. They are far more likely than men to report depression and anxiety.[19]

Women also tend to be cross-addicted, particularly with those drugs whose effects are dangerously magnified when mixed with alcohol. In a 1983 survey by Alcoholics Anonymous, sixty-four percent of their female members under thirty admitted to having been addicted to at least one other drug.[20] One researcher found that as many as forty-two percent of women alcoholics took tranquilizers and nearly twenty-five percent took sleeping pills while drinking. Tragically, but not surprisingly, alcoholic women outnumber men in both completed and attempted suicides.[21]

In addition, women who drink during pregnancy gamble with the possibility that their children may suffer from fetal alcohol syndrome, the third leading cause of mental retardation due to birth defects and the only one that is preventable.[22] The five thousand children born each year with fetal alcohol syndrome show facial disfigurement, poorly formed joints, small head and body size, and genital, kidney, and cardiac defects. An additional thirty-six thousand children a year are born with a range of less severe fetal alcohol effects.[23] Even drinking in light amounts during pregnancy places an unborn child at risk. A 1987 study by the National Institute of Child Health and Human Development indicated that one or two drinks a day increased the risk of urogenital malformations.[24]

The suffering of children born with mental retardation or physical malformations is obvious. The daily suffering these mothers must endure can only be imagined.

Becoming an alcoholic is easy, since alcohol is surely the most accessible of all drugs. Blatant as a colorful wine cooler, it is also hidden in over seven hundred pharmaceutical products. Liquid vitamins, cough medicines and herbal tinctures may be as much as seventy percent alcohol.[25]

Recovering from alcoholism is not easy. As with other sedative-hypnotics, withdrawal from alcohol can be life threatening and should only be attempted under medical supervision. Withdrawal symptoms may include tremulousness, sweating, and dilated pupils. In twenty-five percent of withdrawals, hallucinosis may occur. Delirium tremens—the hallucinatory, disorienting, and terrifying state known as DTs—may occur from two to fourteen days after a woman's last drink.[26]

Tranquilizers or alcohol antagonizing agents such as Antabuse may, in a relatively few cases, be necessary stop-gap measures to sobriety. But, the only cure for alcoholism is abstinence. Any attempt to control the problem by drinking less, by drinking more sensibly, or by drinking just a little now and then is bound to fail.[27]

Women who want to free themselves from alcohol dependence are strongly urged to seek qualified medical advice. Once they leave inpatient or outpatient treatment, some women may need continuing care in a longer-term recovery home. Individual or family counseling, and involvement in a support program with other recovering alcoholics are usually essential for continued sobriety. The advice and encouragement of other women who understand the dynamics of female alcoholism is invaluable. Support programs, such as AA, are available in most communities. One-third of AA members are women, and there are more than six hundred AA women's groups in the United States and Canada.[28]

*   *   *

Jill's Story

Jill is a delicate, red-haired woman in her late thirties. When we met in her office at a midcity hospital, she was wearing a white skirt suit with a green blouse unbuttoned at the neck. Her casual, unharried air was in sharp contrast to the business going on about her—telephone ringing, staff asking directions, and papers needing signing. When these demands were satisfied, she closed the door and told us her story.

I didn't know what an alcoholic was until I was already well on my way. I didn't know drinking could do bad things to you. I didn't know it could be addictive. I didn't see any of that. Nobody ever talked about it.

My father was in the stock market, the manager of a mutual fund. He did regularly have a couple of bourbons with his *Wall Street Journal* when he came home from his daily trip to New York City. But I don't believe he drank alcoholically. So, unlike so many alcoholics I've met who are themselves children of alcoholics, I am not.

There's sort of a feeling that alcoholism is something that wouldn't happen in the Connecticut town I grew up in. People in that town do not go to bars. In fact, I can't think of any bars offhand. They call their liquor stores "package stores" so they don't have to even use the word liquor.

Most people have their package store deliver by the case, so they're all drinking in the privacy of their homes and a lot of them probably dying in the privacy of their homes, from alcoholism.

My first run in with alcohol was when I was fifteen. My parents went somewhere for the evening and I decided to experiment, so I went into their liquor cabinet and poured myself a whole lot of booze, not knowing that you were supposed to mix it and put ice in it. I just poured everything into a glass and drank it and ended up throwing up and blacking out. From my very first drink I could never handle it. I never knew when to stop.

When my parents came home a few hours later, they found their darling daughter passed out in the bathroom. I was very sick and vowed the next day I would never touch it again. And I never did, for about another two years.

My parents made me go to an all-girls private high school, much against my will. I hated it and built up four years of resentment about all the fun and parties I was missing. What kept me going was my vow that I would make up for those four years as soon as I got to college.

In my senior year, when I was seventeen, I started dating seriously. The guy was a year older than I and had already started college. The two of us went to parties and drank *a lot*. For instance, we'd go to the drive-in with another couple. They'd take a six-pack of beer *between* them to last through two movies. We would take a six-pack of beer for *each* one of us. There was a difference in tolerance and we would make little jokes about drinking more than the other people and say that they couldn't hold it and weren't we terrific, not knowing that this is one of the very first signs of alcoholism—to be able to hold a lot of booze and not show it.

I kept dating the same guy when I went away to Cedar College, the very good, well-respected Ivy League school that gives you lots of social status. Nice girls went there, and even if people noticed that I came back from the dorm drunk—which I'm sure they did—or that I stayed out after curfew—which I'm sure they did—it was considered general college fun and not an alcohol problem, because nice girls who go to Cedar College don't become alcoholics.

It went without saying that drinking would go on throughout the weekend. We went to dances and drank. We structured our events around alcohol. If you want to have fun, you want to be where alcohol is. We hardly ever did anything that did not involve alcohol.

It continued like that all the way through college. It never interfered with my grades, because I was only doing it on weekends. And, again, it looked very normal and acceptable—that's what all college kids do.

But after college was over, those other college kids were expected to grow up, settle down, become responsible, get good jobs and generally handle their lives. What happened in my case was, when my four years in college were over, I found myself terrified of doing any of those things. Part of me never grew up and did not want to be responsible. In fact, I was terrified of going out into the world and taking care of myself. I somehow never developed that ego strength that enables most kids to make their way on their own. I just wanted to keep partying.

"We surrounded ourselves with people who drank."

So when it came time to graduate, my best idea was to go on and get some more school and a master's degree. Of course, that's a very socially acceptable thing to do. It looked real good. My parents were certainly willing to pay for it. But the real reason I was doing it was because I was too scared to do anything else.

This was in 1966. I entered Benchley University to get my master's degree in social work. I was scared to death going to a brand new school where I didn't know anybody. I didn't have a lot of social skills. I really didn't know how to relate to people—I was very shy. But I knew that if I had a couple of drinks in me, I would be fine.

On the very first day at the university, when class was over, I started talking to one of the guys in my class, and he casually said, "How would you like to go out for a beer?" And I said I thought that would be a fine idea. I was looking for a socially accepted way to get back into drinking again. We ended up going to a bar.

If you're not an alcoholic, I don't know how to tell you this other than to say, I think there is some kind of invisible antenna whereby alcoholics can find each other. We sat there and drank for three hours and I knew in my heart this man drank like I did.

And that's how it works with alcoholic women. We seek out other people, particularly men, who drink like we do because then we don't have to feel guilty about our alcohol consumption. We don't have to worry about someone looking at us funny and saying, "Boy, you're certainly drinking a lot." Because someone else who's doing the same is not going to say that to me. In fact, he's not going to say anything at all. And that's how we get ourselves into crazy relationships that we have a hell of a time getting out of and which cause us to drink even more. So, Alan and I became inseparable. We went to the same classes and spent most of our time together.

He decided he was in love with me. I knew I wasn't really in love with him, but the relationship was so easy. There was never any question about drinking.

We stayed together for the two years we were at Benchley getting our master's degrees. My attention to my studies was going down at this point. I was living on my own and could drink any time I wanted to. So, the disease progressed a little bit. Of course, I didn't know I had a disease.

We surrounded ourselves with people who drank like we did. I can remember distinctly at this point changing friends, turning away from the people who didn't like to drink, feeling uncomfortable around them. In order to make that okay, I made them, in my mind, sticks-in-the-mud. They didn't like to have fun. They didn't know how to party. They were boring. They were too intellectual. They liked to study all the time.

It was 1968 when it came time to graduate. Alan told me he loved me and wanted to get married. He asked me to marry him when he graduated.

I knew in my heart of hearts I didn't love this man and marrying him would be an extreme disservice to us both. On the other hand, I thought, if I marry him, he will probably not get drafted to Vietnam and we'd have a good time drinking together and I wouldn't have to interrupt my partying. I was still terrified of being by myself, and here was someone who wanted to be with me and drink with me. It all seemed to work out into a nice neat package.

I can remember walking down the aisle with this man thinking, "I don't love him. What am I doing? You're making a mistake. You're going to hurt him. You're going to hurt yourself. This is not going to work." But I did it anyway.

"On a typical night we both went into blackouts."

I got very drunk at the reception so I wouldn't have to think about what I had just done and we had a lovely honeymoon in Montreal at the World's Fair.

To insure that he didn't have to go to Vietnam, we went into VISTA, Volunteers in Service to America, which at that time was like a domestic Peace Corps. It was called alternative service. We moved to the slums of Detroit, into an apartment above a butcher shop. We didn't go out to a pub anymore. Instead we started going to the grocery store and picking up a fifth of bourbon every night. We'd say, here's what we're going to have for dinner—a steak, baked potato, salad—and then his arm or my arm just reached as the basket passed the liquor section and grabbed the bottle and we took it home and killed it.

I knew deep down this was not normal drinking, and I'm sure he did too. But by this time we had developed the No-Talk Rule. We never talked about it. We got loaded every night, and got up every morning with a hangover and went to work. I started very much looking forward to five o'clock when we could do it all over again.

On a typical night, we both went into a blackout. Most normal drinkers, if they had a blackout, would be horrified and just wouldn't drink again. Alcoholic drinkers try to push out of their minds the fact that they can't remember a whole part of the evening before.

That's what happened to me. We'd say things to each other and the next morning wake up and not know what we had said. If one person is going to black out, it's confusing enough in a relationship. But if both people are in a blackout, it's crazy.

This went on for two years. By this time I was definitely psychologically hooked. I had to have that booze every night. Physically I was starting to feel real bad. The disease of alcoholism progresses faster in women than in men and I started to feel sick. The hangovers started to get to me.

Now, the biggest part of the disease of alcohol is denial and rationalization. I needed something or someone to blame for what was happening to me and it was real easy to blame him. I convinced myself, with my alcoholic thinking, that I never drank like this until I got hooked up with this guy and that maybe it would be a good idea if we weren't together anymore.

I told him I was very unhappy with him. We separated for a while and had many talks about whether or not we should get back together. We always had these talks in a bar. We'd have martinis and discuss what our problems were and why our marriage wasn't working. We never got anywhere. Finally, he agreed to give me a divorce.

"I started doing all the things alcoholics do."

Here was my best plan: leave Detroit, start a new life in brand new, sunny Southern California. I had heard it was wonderful and I very much wanted to go there. My dad had some business dealing with a company in San Diego and he got me a job with them. I thought, "Well, gee, this sounds interesting. A change of pace."

I had become involved, after my divorce in Detroit, with another man and he wanted to come out with me. That was music to my ears, because as always, I was terrified of being alone.

So I moved to San Diego in 1971 and got a house. I had this nice easy job that my father had set up for me working for a real estate investment trust, working under the controller, helping him to keep track of all the millions of dollars this trust had loaned out all over the country. It was real easy. My general level of functioning had gone down a lot due to the alcohol and that was all I was capable of at that point.

I stayed in that job for three years and my life started to get miserable. My body really wanted that drink at five o'clock. This was the onset of real physical addiction. I would get into my little car and speed home at five o'clock to get to the liquor store.

I started doing all the things alcoholics do. I went to one liquor store one night, then another the next night. I didn't want anyone to know how much I was drinking. I'd try to keep track of what store I went to what night so I didn't blow it and go to the same store twice in a row.

I started hiding my bottles in other people's trash cans because I didn't want anyone to know the whole garbage can was filled with bottles.

I switched from one thing to another. I thought, "This hard stuff is not very good for me. I think I'll drink just wine." For three years I just drank Gallo wine. Every night. A *lot* of Gallo wine.

"I was totally losing control over my life."

My life started to get very, very depressing. I was always depressed. I was very isolated. By this time I was afraid to make a lot of new friends because I didn't want anyone to know how much I was drinking. I thought moving to California would solve my drinking problem, and all my other problems. And I found out very quickly that wasn't so.

So here I am. I'm divorced, in a strange town, in a job I'm not at all trained for and living with a guy that, again, I didn't really want to have a permanent relationship with and he was pressuring me to do that.

He was not an alcoholic. He was very much the opposite. He was very much against my drinking. He saw what it was doing to me; he really cared about me. He did all of the things that people who live with alcoholics do. He would try to dissuade me from going to the liquor store. When that didn't work, he went for me. He bought all my booze for me. Poor guy. I really gave him hell. He just kind of threw up his hands and let me drink. And drink I did. Lots.

I started to feel worse and worse in the morning. By this time it was real obvious to me I had a definite alcohol problem. But I felt so ashamed and so embarrassed and all the things that alcoholics feel, particularly women. In moments of clarity I would look at myself in the mirror and say, "What is happening to you? You have six years of college, you're doing a dumb job, you have no friends, you feel bad about yourself, your life is not the way you want it to be. What's wrong here?"

But because of my screwed-up thinking and my low self-esteem, it was easier just to keep drinking. You see, when you're drunk, you don't have to think about this stuff because you're all numbed out.

I was miserable and very afraid. I didn't know what to do. I felt I had gotten myself into a trap and I didn't know how to get out. And this was a worse trap than the one in Detroit. I was totally losing control over my life. I wanted to quit the job but didn't know what else to do and needed the money. My parents couldn't help because I was writing them letters that everything was fine.

I knew in my heart of hearts that alcohol was the problem, but I did not know what to do. I was addicted and I *could not stop*. I could not see how to stop. I couldn't tell anybody about it. I was ashamed. I hated myself. That went on for three years.

Finally, one night the phone rang and it was my ex-husband, calling from Ohio, where he was living. He was kind of loaded and I was kind of loaded, and he said, "How are you doing?" I said,

"Not so good." He asked, "Would you like to try again? I miss you." And I said, "This is the answer to my prayers. Sure!" So I used him again, only this time it worked out a little differently.

I said goodbye to the guy I had been living with and driving crazy for the last three years. Alan came out to California and packed up all my stuff. Driving back to Ohio, we made an agreement that we wouldn't get remarried, but at least we would try living together for awhile.

Now in the three years we hadn't seen each other, his drinking had stayed the same. He was still what you call a "functioning alcoholic." But I had started going down, like a rock. I was shaking in the morning now, and getting sick.

When we were back in Ohio, Alan made a major mistake. He said to me, "Sounds like you've had a pretty rough three years. Why don't you take the summer off?" That was music to my ears.

While he was at work, I watched soap operas and drank beer all day. So now I was drinking in the daytime *and* nighttime.

Needless to say, after a few months of coming home every night from work and finding his ex-wife half in the bag, Alan was not thrilled. The arguing started again. Finally, he got disgusted and said, "You've got to leave."

"I flipped out and took a knife from the kitchen."

His mother came out and packed up all my stuff. She took me to the airport and she said, "We just don't want you in our son's life anymore. You're very sick. You need help." Of course, they never told me where to go to get it.

Back in California I met another man. I thought, "If I marry him, I could straighten up, stop drinking and my problems would be over." He thought he could save me from my drinking. We both thought the power of love could overcome this little drinking problem.

I moved in with him on a trial basis and promised him I'd stop drinking. But I couldn't. Every day he went to work and I'd try so hard not to drink and every day I'd fail. I'd go down to the local store and buy some beer and some wine and come home and drink. I just hated myself every day.

It was the worst pain I ever felt in my life because I wanted so badly to straighten up. By this time, I was physically and emotionally addicted and I couldn't.

One night he finally snapped and said, "This is ridiculous. I'm not going to marry you. You can't straighten out. I can't handle this anymore. You've got to get out of here."

He called up my parents in Connecticut and told them, "I can't marry your daughter. She's an alcoholic. You deal with her. I've had it." And that's how my parents found out that I was an alcoholic.

I flipped out and took a knife from the kitchen, ran into the bathroom and cut my wrists. We had to go to the emergency room. I really did want to die because I was so miserable, I couldn't see going on another day. But I ended up going to my parents' house.

They were sure that if I stayed with them for three months and didn't drink, I'd be fine. They didn't understand anything about alcoholism, and neither did I.

After a month, they started giving me a cocktail with them before dinner. Neither one of us knew that one drink is what gets you drunk. I had the drink, then waited till they went to bed and then I got into the liquor. They ended up taking the liquor out of their house and putting it in a locked suitcase in the garage so I wouldn't get at it.

That's when they finally figured out that maybe their darling little daughter really *did* have an alcohol problem. But they didn't know what to do. Nobody knew.

"I didn't want anybody to see what I had become."

I felt so bad because I knew I was hurting my parents and I couldn't stop. I was just doing what every alcoholic does: hurting the people who were closest to me in my life.

After the ninety days, I told them I had to go back to California to find my own answer to my life. "I appreciate what you've done," I said, "but you can't babysit me forever."

Back in California, I vowed that either something from the blue was going to come and save me or I was going to end up drinking myself to death.

Every day I'd go to the store, get my wine and watch the damn soap operas all day long. That was my only connection to the world. My other was the radio. I'd listen to the radio and I'd start calling disc jockeys and start talking to them. A couple of them ended up coming over to my house and we'd party and I'd sleep with them. I thought I was really in great shape. I was sleeping with disc jockeys. I did that for more than two years. But I didn't have a whole lot of sex those last two years, because I wanted to be alone.

By this time I was really in the very late chronic stages to where eating wasn't fun anymore, so I'd go several days without eating.

When I woke up I would have grapefruit juice and wine for breakfast. Then I'd have some beer or wine for lunch. And there wasn't anyone to watch after me. They were all gone by now. With the exception of some very old friends, I was by myself, totally isolated, determined to shut myself off from the world because I didn't want anybody to see what I had become.

I started to get sick, of course, from not eating and from the effects of the alcohol. This was when I started going to hospitals. About every six months or so, I'd get so sick, a friend of mine would come over and say, "Well, it looks like it's time to take you to the hospital again." And I'd get carted off.

With no insurance, one does not get treated for alcohol. So I ended up in psycho wards, which are set up to treat mental disorders, usually with medication. I'd go to one hospital, get filled with Valium, then a few months later I'd go to another. By this time, I thought, "Well, I keep landing in psycho wards, so I must be crazy. That's why I drink so much and that's the problem."

The psychiatrists I saw don't know anything about alcoholism. They gave me Antabuse, the drug that makes you throw up when you drink. Their solution to my drinking problem was, "Don't drink and take Antabuse." Needless to say, I figured out that if you don't take the Antabuse, you can drink.

"They took me to my first AA meeting."

Finally, I ended up getting a citation for drunk driving. That was part of reaching my bottom, because it was so humiliating. I couldn't imagine this nice social worker from an upper middle-class Connecticut family being handcuffed, put in the back of a police car and taken downtown to jail. It was so demoralizing to me. One of my drinking buddies came and got me out after four hours. That's what they call a quick release program but four hours is plenty!

It finally began to dawn on me, maybe I was going to die from this disease. Maybe it was really happening to me. No one was going to come along and rescue me this time. So, when the last friend I had left in the world came over and said, "I think you need treatment for alcoholism," something clicked in my head. I said, "Okay, let's go." And suddenly she called my parents.

This friend explained to my parents that with no insurance I couldn't get the help I needed and that if they could send the money to get me to an alcohol treatment program, my chances of getting well were really good. And the miracle of miracles happened and that's the way it worked.

My parents sent the money and this friend carted me off to Carlyle Hill Hospital.

I only vaguely remember going in at all. I'm sure I had to have help walking in. I don't remember signing papers. I was probably not capable of doing that either. This is the college graduate with a master's. Couldn't walk, couldn't talk, couldn't eat. Not functional. I don't know how close to dying I really was. But I felt I was.

Then they took me to my first AA meeting. I'll never forget it as long as I live because I always thought I was the only person who ever did any of those alcoholic things—the only person who hid bottles, who went to different liquor stores, who didn't eat for days at a time, the only person who watched soap operas and drank all day. I thought I was the worst of the worst and the lowest of the low.

But these people had done all the same things and and were laughing about them. They weren't ashamed. They were happy people. I thought, "Wow, there's something going on here. There is hope—there is hope." I got hope from that first meeting.

I first heard there that I had a disease. I wasn't a bad person and it wasn't Jill who had done all the bad things, it was the disease doing those things. If I followed the program they laid out for me, I could be sober, too, and wouldn't have to do any of those things anymore. I might even be a happy person again, which I had long since given up on. I started to cry. Because I felt I had come home.

I just kept going back to those meetings. And hope got bigger and bigger and bigger. And pretty soon I started eating again, and feeling good again.

"I knew that it was going to work out."

I learned at meetings that, if I just stayed away from that first drink, I would be okay, because it's the first drink that gets you drunk. That was a big revelation to me. All these years I'd been trying to drink like a lady, like a normal drinker. Have those two beers and leave the bar. Have those two drinks and leave the party. It never worked. I couldn't understand it. Then I figured out what the disease was all about. It's about the first drink. Once you have the first one, forget it. It's all over. If you're an alcoholic.

So I had no trouble taking Step One, admitting I was powerless over alcohol and my life was unmanageable. God, I was practically dead. How unmanageable can you get?

I'd been evicted from my last apartment when I entered the treatment program. Thank God for my dad, who kept sending me money, kept believing in me, even after all the crazy things I did. I took the money and I put a down payment on a new apartment. This was going to be my first sober apartment. I got out of the hospital and went to the apartment and I made myself a rule. There will be no booze in this apartment! Ever! And I haven't broken it to this day. That's one of the things I do to keep sober. I do not keep alcohol in my house.

I didn't do a whole lot the first year, because it took me a full year just to learn how to live all over again. I learned how to drive sober. I learned how to go to the grocery store and shop without having the cart go in the liquor section. I learned how to make new friends, and most of them were in AA.

Things started getting better and better. My self-confidence came back a little bit.

One day I was at a meeting and heard this woman speak of a college program for people who wanted to be counselors in alcoholism. I had been wondering, now that I'd been given my life back, what the heck was I going to do with it? I was so grateful for what I'd been given through AA, I wanted to give some back. I thought, "This could be great." I could take my social work skills, learn counseling skills about alcoholism, put them all together and go work in the field. And that's just what I did!

By the time I got out of the counseling program, I was two years sober. I had a lot of friends. I had a good solid foundation for sobriety through AA, and I just turned my future over to a higher power. I knew that, somehow or other, it was going to work out. I had hope. I had built up, gradually, this faith that, as self-destructive as I had been, as willful and immature, this higher power wanted me to live, otherwise I would never have gotten to Carlyle Hill Hospital.

Lo and behold, a week after I got out of this program, a job opened up in a women's recovery home called Turn About and I went to work there. I began to realize how incredible the problems of alcoholic women are. Not that men don't have problems, but women will stand by their alcoholic men. Most men don't stand by their women. So by the time women get to a place like Turn About, everyone has deserted them. And most of them have no job skills. Or any knowledge about how to go out and make it in the world. Because men are taught from day one that someday you're going to grow up to be a man and you've got to go out there and make your own living and you've got to do all those aggressive things. Women are just supposed to be good mommies and take care of the kids and a man will take care of them.

I saw at Turn About that one of the main blocks for women who are alcoholics is that they know, if they ever get sober they're going to have some problems to face and they can't handle thinking about it. They can't handle going out there and being in charge of their own lives.

"If I did it, you can do it."

After I had been at Turn About for two years, the most prestigious hospital treatment program around called and asked me if I wanted to work there. The people at Turn About encouraged me to take that big step, and I worked at that hospital for a year and a half and it was wonderful.

One day, I was looking at the want ads in the paper and saw an ad for a counselor at Carlyle Hill. That was the very hospital, the very program, where I had gotten sober! I thought, "Why not?" I applied for the job and got it.

I worked at Carlyle Hill for a year when my boss, the man who ran the entire program, left. I applied for the job and, lo and behold, I got it! And that's where I've been ever since, in charge of the very program that I entered as a total wreck not so long ago.

I see women who are like what I was coming in and out of that program all the time. I see the women who are lost and frightened. It is such a blessing to sit down and hold someone's hand and say, "If I did it, you can do it." And they look at me and say, "You were an alcoholic?" And I say, "Just a little while ago, I was sitting on this very same bed."

3

Valium
Melanie's Story

Five Billion Doses Yearly

Although they are officially classified as minor tranquilizers, the Valium-family drugs are clearly in the major leagues when it comes to lethality. In 1984, they were cited in an estimated fifty thousand incidents that ended in emergency room treatment. Sixty percent of these incidents involved women. In 1984 Valium-like drugs were a factor in over six hundred female drug deaths.[1]

But these figures barely hint at the true extent of Valium use and abuse. The Drug Abuse Warning Network estimates that ten million Americans have used Valium for nonmedical purposes at some point in their lives. Four million have done so in the past year alone.[2]

Valium has become infamous as the most indiscriminately prescribed psychoactive drug in history. Ninety-seven percent of all family doctors and internists prescribe it.[3] It is most commonly given as a muscle relaxant, tranquilizer or sleep aid, but is sometimes given *to fight fatigue*. Sixty-five percent of Valium users are women.[4] As Liza Minnelli put it, "They throw it at you like candy."

Each year Americans take more than *five billion* medically approved doses of Valium and Valium-like tranquilizers.[5] The enormous number of prescriptions—seventy million per year—prompted the American Medical Association to warn doctors against overprescribing.[6,7] Despite this, studies indicate that three-fourths of all prescriptions are being written for conditions inconsistent with the approved use of these drugs.[8]

As a Schedule IV drug, a Valium prescription can be renewed up to five times within six months. The staggering quantities of the drug which someone may be consuming under doctor's orders has given some researchers pause. In 1981, a doctor at Mt. Sinai Hospital in New York City tested more than two hundred anxiety-ridden patients, giving some Valium and some placebos. After the first week of treatment, the placebo proved as effective as Valium. Anyone taking Valium for more than a week, this study seems to say, might just as well be taking sugar pills.[9]

Valium is a member of the benzodiazepine (BZP) family, a class of minor tranquilizers that now includes, among many others, Ativan, Centrax, Dalmane, Halcion, Librium, Paxipam, Restoril, Serax, Sereen, Tranxene, Verstran, and Xanax. A full list of all the BZPs would read something like the phone book of a small town. The Roche Company, Valium's creator, estimates there are *seven hundred* Valium imitations.[10] But despite their different sizes, shapes, colors, and packaging, all the BZPs are near clones, and what is said about one can be said about all.

Perhaps more than any other substance, the BZPs are a woman's drug. In their book, *Beyond Valium*, authors Rosenblatt and Dodson recount the telling story of an executive at Roche who was plagued with a "virago" of a mother-in-law. Looking to cure his "mother-in-law-itis," the man got some Librium the lab was working on and told the woman it was a new drug for "sensitive temperaments." The woman was fooled by this "innocuous sugges-tion" and took some pills. Instantly, she was a changed woman, no longer "irritable and cranky." A shrew had been tamed. As Rosenblatt and Dodson conclude, "In one fell swoop the executive saved his home life and put the final zing into Roche's promotional efforts."[11]

This next step in the BZP's ascendancy was an elaborate and costly ad campaign that cleverly zeroed in on women as its prime market. Full page ads in medical journals pictured young co-eds nervously clutching their books, harried housewives surrounded by a jail of brooms and mops, and mothers dejectedly sitting at school functions. There was nothing wrong with them that a couple of pills couldn't cure. As one woman observed, "A woman's emotional problems are usually treated as a Valium deficiency."

Although women routinely take the Valium-family drugs for symptoms that include anxiety, fatigue, tension, depression, and insomnia, among their observed side effects are: anxiety, fatigue, tension, depression and insomnia. This paradox prompted one doctor to ask: "What am I supposed to do if I prescribe it and the symptoms continue? Stop the drug or double the dose?"[12]

All the Valium users we spoke with "cured" their side effects by doubling the dose. One woman called this "fighting Valium with Valium."

Many of us continue to believe that a powerful drug like Valium must surely be safe at sensible dose levels. But in testimony before a U.S. Senate subcommittee, one doctor stated that seventy-five to eighty percent of people taking "normal-range doses" of the Valium drugs have impaired intellectual functioning. Some studies have indicated that such symptoms can be observed after only *one* dose of Valium. Other researchers have reported that Valium and Librium may cause permanent brain damage.[13]

Another misconception about the BZPs is that they are basically nonaddictive. Women who have been taking them for months or years are thought to suffer from a medical or emotional condition, not a drug problem. One team of researchers found that doctors who first judged a group of people as drug-dependent later softened their opinion when told the drug in question was Valium.[14]

The users of tranquilizers have a different perspective. In a 1976 study of fifty Valium users, twenty-four people tried to stop using and couldn't. Twenty-three others did stop and suffered withdrawal symptoms.[15] In 1980, more than seven thousand people entered treatment centers because of tranquilizer addiction. More than forty-five hundred were seeking help from drugs for the first time.[16] In that same year, estimates of those being treated by private doctors for BZP withdrawal ran as high as twenty thousand.[17]

The number of people hooked on the Valium-like drugs is estimated to be at least one and a half million.[18] The majority of them are women.[19] And many of them won't see the hold Valium has over them until they stop taking their pills. Withdrawal symptoms, which almost always take three to five days to appear, and sometimes as many as ten days, can include pain, muscle cramps, tremors, headaches, anxiety, nausea, and depression. Convulsions and loss of memory can also occur. Some former addicts say kicking this supposedly nonaddictive family of drugs is harder than kicking heroin. Saying goodbye to Valium and its cousins is an act of strength that requires expert guidance and knowledgeable care.

While use of the BZPs has steadily declined over the past ten years, Valium is still the top-selling psychoactive drug in America. A spokesperson for Hoffman-LaRoche reported that in 1984 twenty-five million prescriptions were written for Valium alone.[20] And now that the patent for Valium has expired, we may expect other drug companies to introduce their own generic form, bringing down prices, boosting sales.

In our interviews for this book, Valium was mentioned more than any other drug. One amphetamine abuser told us, "It isn't a question of *whether* you'll take Valium, but *when*." Several women who were diagnosed as using too much alcohol were given Valium in its stead, a procedure that one doctor likened to treating lung cancer with cigarettes. "Your patients don't get better," another doctor has said, "they just *smell* better."[21]

Although we were not dedicated users, we usually had some Valium around. We used it to come down from psychedelics or coke, or to smooth things out after a bad day. For us, Valium was like a side order that seemed to go well with any number of main courses. But even we felt its bite, because unlike other drugs which cause serious harm to long-time or mega-dose users, Valium shows its downside to even "normal" users.

What is needed to counteract the unrelenting advertising and propaganda campaign waged on Valium's behalf is an equally dedicated education effort. The story that follows is one step in peeling off the mask of tranquility that hides the Valium-family grimace. Melanie's story is compelling for another reason: she is a survivor of incest.

* * *

Melanie's Story

Melanie is a vivacious woman in her midthirties with black curly hair. She combines strength and softness in an appealing way. She is head of public relations for the chemical dependency unit of a large hospital. We interviewed her in her pleasantly decorated home, where she lives with her husband and her two teen-age daughters. She has been clean and sober for eight years.

My dad started putting the make on me when I was twelve. He always waited until my mother left the house, so as soon as I knew she was going, I numbed out. I just turned off and got real passive. There was never any actual penetration, but he'd touch me and feel me a lot. I knew what he was doing was bad, but he said if I told my mother, she would probably leave him. So I felt the responsibility and the guilt and all that stuff.

He came from a background of abuse and, as you know, it gets passed down. I heard him tell stories about his father whipping him with a branch with thorns left on it. He was the oldest of eight children, five of whom were alcoholics and I suspect there was incest between him and some of his sisters.

On my mother's side, her father and oldest brother died of alcoholism, and she's got a young brother currently dying of it. Between both sides of the family, I have about forty cousins and I would say a lot of them are alcoholic or have a problem with drugs. My mother and father were both Bible-carrying fundamentalists.

During my teen years I was attractive and boys liked me. When I started to date, I was very open and gregarious if I was in a group, but when I was alone with a boy I got terrified. I couldn't talk and I got real, real uncomfortable, until I met Dan. I felt safe with him and we started going together in my junior year.

By my senior year, my father had gotten really bad. I was starring in the spring musical and spending a lot of time at rehearsals. One night my father said I'd been too busy and had to quit the play and said, "You can't go out for the rest of the year." I was so terrified of him that I had never spoken back. But that night, maybe because Dan was there, I shouted, "I don't care what you say, I'm going to finish what I started." He kicked me up against the wall and almost killed me. Dan had to lift him off me. My eyes were black. My teeth had gone through my lip. And that was just for talking back to him.

Two months later I graduated from high school and married Dan. I married to get out. Period. I remember thinking as I walked down the aisle that I didn't love him and that I was marrying for all the wrong reasons. His family had money so I knew I would be well taken care of. Well, maybe I could learn to love him.

"Then I got addicted to being up."

Three months into marriage, I had my first drink. Dan had fixed these exotic drinks with some Bacardi 180-proof rum in an Osterizer we had gotten as a wedding present. We had another couple over and the woman confided that her husband was a real pervert. When I got drunk, I told him I thought he was a jackass and should leave his wife alone. At this point, Dan started handing me straight booze and I drank it down. Most people would have passed out but I kept going till three in the morning. I was real crazy. I was crying. All these feelings were coming up. This was the start of how I'd react to alcohol, lots and lots of crying and anger and what I call acting out. It was the most godawful scene. But I loved the way I felt when I drank, and I loved the way it tasted. Finally, I got violently ill.

The next day my mother came over and found me lying on the bathroom floor. I told her I had food poisoning. I didn't drink after that for a couple of years—I was scared to death of it. When I started again, I just drank beer because I could better control how drunk I got.

In the beginning there were some good years. We always lived in big houses with swimming pools in the nicest parts of suburbia and drove nice cars. We had race boats and spent a lot time down at the Colorado River. In the early years we kept everything relatively normal at home but we'd go down to the Colorado River to party and just raise hell. I mean, we'd start drinking on the way down and didn't sober up for days.

It wasn't too long before I realized my husband was an alcoholic, and it wasn't too long before the abuse started. At first he was only emotionally abusive, like never acknowledging anything I did. Maybe he was afraid if he said, "You did a good job," or "I like who you are," I would get a big head and leave him.

After I had my first child I started using speed. I had gained maybe ten pounds and I went down to Dr. Quack and for seven or eight bucks I got some amphetamines and diuretics and within a few weeks I lost the weight. Then I got addicted to being up, even when I didn't need to lose weight. I had years and years of speed use, always from Dr. Quack and an OBGYN I went to when I was having a real difficult time carrying my second baby. He gave me as much amphetamine as I wanted. We also had some friends who sold us jars of Bennies. I probably used speed off and on for about fifteen to twenty years.

"What started out as a transference turned into an affair."

When my children were small I felt real content, but when they got to be about three years old, I started feeling restless and antsy and noticed a lot of things missing in the marriage. So I'd have another baby and start the process all over again. But I wasn't in love with my husband, he didn't turn me on, and I was getting infatuated with other men. I had read *The Sensuous Woman* and decided, "Oh, my God, I'm not orgasmic, what am I going to do, my life is over." And that spurred me on to therapy.

My first therapist was one of these brilliant people who changes careers every five years, going from airline pilot to ordained Episcopalian minister to clinical psychologist. At the time I was thirty-two, he was pushing fifty. I remember telling him that I thought I might be an alcoholic. But whatever he thought an alcoholic looked like, I didn't fit the picture. He was the first person to prescribe Valium for me, to get me to sleep at night after I had been up all day on speed. I just kind of drifted into solid sedatives that way.

He felt if I could get angry at him I'd let go some of the rage that I had for my dad. But what started out as a transference turned into an affair. He kept saying, "Trust me, this is what we need to do." It set me back light years.

I left him and found my way to another psychiatrist who diagnosed me as manic-depressive and added Elavil to my Valium.

" 'Melanie, what on your application is true?' "

My husband's alcoholism had progressed and by now he was physically abusive. A couple of times he damned near killed me. One day he came upstairs and he said, "Somebody broke into the house last night and demolished our living room." "That somebody is you," I said. He had wrecked the living room and couldn't remember. I'd get violent, too, and those last few years were just awful.

After fifteen years of marriage and three kids, we broke up. Until that time, I had never worked, other than a little direct sales; he had always taken care of me. I didn't even know how to balance a checkbook. When I moved out I rented a grandiose apartment I couldn't afford with lemon-yellow carpeting. He wasn't going to help me with much money so I got a job as a teacher's aide with emotionally handicapped kids making about five bucks an hour.

After a couple of months, I freaked. I just collapsed. I had . . . not really a breakdown. I think it was a combination of too much drinking and too much speed. My psychiatrist sent me to a regular mental hospital to dry out and I stayed for five months, basket weaving and having a blast. I'd sit around the pool at Happy Dale Sanatorium, as I called it, and smoke dope. When staff came over I'd say, "What are you going to do, lock me up?" I did everything I wasn't supposed to. It was a wild time.

One day I was sitting there thinking, everyone says I can't make it without my husband. So I asked my doctor to let me go out for some job interviews. "What are you going to do?" he asked. "You've hardly ever worked." And I said, "I'm going to go interview for some sales jobs." He said, "Okay, Melanie, go for it."

I was interviewed by a very large manufacturer of business forms, and gave my mother's telephone number as my home phone. They'd call her to say, "We need Melanie to come back for another interview." She'd call me at the mental hospital and I'd call them back for another appointment. After weeks of calls and interviews I walked in and said, "I'd really like to work here but I've been offered another job." The head of personnel said, "Don't do anything till you talk to me. I'll get back to you tonight." So he finally hired me.

I got out of the hospital on a Friday and showed up for work the following Monday, on Elavil, Valium and stimulants. I'm in an office with thirty-three salesmen who have never worked with a woman in their lives. I had a real plush office with a gorgeous view and I was making incredible money for a woman in 1973, plus car allowance, plus commission. I thought, "This is not bad, the kid's done okay for herself." The qualifications for this job were two years' recent sales experience and a marketing degree. I didn't even know how to answer a phone with lights and buttons on it.

A few days later, the personnel guy who hired me comes into my office with his veins sticking out of his neck. He had the reputation of being this wonderful interviewer who never hired anyone but the most capable people. He looks at me and says, "Melanie, what on your application is true?" And I answer, "My name, my sex, and my social security number." He says, "You've made me look like a damn fool. I never want to see you again." I walked out of the office thinking, "Well, win some, lose some."

The next morning he called me up and asked me to come back to work. He said he had never in his life been conned like that and if I could con him, I could sell anything. For the next year he personally trained me. Three years later I was one of the company's top five salespeople. The very last order I wrote for them was over a million and a half dollars. It was the largest single order they ever placed.

"I took a couple of hundred Valium."

After I'd been there a while, the personnel head called and said, "Block out the next two weekends. We're going to Palm Springs." I said, "You must be crazy. You're married." He said, "That doesn't matter. I'll pick you up Friday night." "I'm not available," I said and hung up on him. Friday night he walked into my bedroom, took stuff out of my drawers, put it in a suitcase, put a purse over my shoulder and off we went to Palm Springs. He was one of those very, very strong men, maybe the first man I really cared about. We ended up having an affair; his wife found out and they divorced.

Throughout this time I drank and used. Sometimes I was fine, other times I got so depressed, feeling guilty that I had been a bad mother and a bad wife. I never looked at my husband as part of the problem. I always thought it was my problem, my fault, I did it. If I'd only be different, if I could only straighten out everything would be fine. And I was hurting everybody. Despite the fact that I was so successful in my job, making more money than I'd seen in my entire life, I was in a lot of pain most of the time and becoming suicidal.

One night I took a couple of hundred Valium and bottles of aspirins and any other pill I found—if it was a pill, I took it. My husband had just picked up the girls for the weekend. He drove away and after fifteen minutes he remembered that he hadn't taken the kids' jackets. He came back and found everything locked up and my car outside. When I didn't answer his knocking, he went up to the second-story balcony, broke a plate glass door and got me to the hospital in time. They pumped my stomach and sent me right back home. I was all swollen up. My eyes had swollen shut. I had a lot of water retention for a few days. If you ever want to commit suicide, Valium isn't the way.

By this time my mom and dad had gotten real sick of all the trauma, the depression, the totaled cars. They loved my husband and felt that if I would only straighten out and be Donna Reed everything would be fine. They had no idea what was wrong with me. They certainly didn't know it was alcoholism and addiction. In fact my mother used to give me a lot of the pills. She'd buy Valium by the hundreds and was always quite willing to share her supply.

I went back to my husband after a year's separation thinking it was safe there and a place I could hide. Within two days I knew I had made a mistake. I looked around this great big house and thought, "Nothing's changed. The house hasn't changed, he hasn't changed, and yet I *have* changed."

That's when I really started hitting it. I had an expense account at work and was expected to take customers out to drink. When I came back to the office bombed, no one said anything, everyone thought it was funny. I drank and smoked dope with the salesmen.

Then my psychiatrist finally saw some daylight and sent me to AA. I went to my first meeting, in 1973, with a pocketful of Valium and speed.

"I used AA to hide in."

I connected with those people immediately and started hanging out at a little clubhouse with the real down-and-outers in AA, straight off skid row. I'd go in there and they'd love me to death. It was like being warmed by a great big fire. I just loved those people and I loved that club. I was loaded on the pills but I didn't drink. My husband was still drinking so he fought against my attempt to quit.

I'd work all day, then hang out at the AA club and meetings and come home at midnight. I used AA to hide in—AA was really like a drug. It kept me from having to go home and deal with my husband. The only time I ever saw him was on weekends. I wasn't spending any time with the kids. I did this for several years. My husband kept saying, "I think you need to be home with the kids; they're at the age when they need you home. . . ." Finally, it was easier to give in. I just got worn down and resigned from the job. I had loved that job. It's very hard after you've done something like that and acquired a measure of success to go back to baking cookies.

We moved to a bigger house in a very affluent neighborhood, complete with Jacuzzi and swimming pool. I was driving a Jag XJ12. And I'd sit in the house thinking about how to do myself in so it wouldn't be real messy and the kids wouldn't know it was suicide.

Meanwhile, because I wasn't drinking, I was getting stronger and more aware of my situation. My husband was doing some strange things, like buying other businesses without telling me. We were getting ready to build a really grandiose five-thousand-square-foot house on the knob of a hill and yet collection agencies were coming around because he wasn't paying the monthly bills. For the first time I realized maybe I wasn't the only family sickie. Until then I had figured, since my alcoholism was so much worse, he wasn't an alcoholic. His was more controlled.

We were just numbed out to each other. Then one night in a fit of anger he brought up the time years ago when I had an affair with his best friend, and said, "I've never forgiven you for what you've done. I've hated you ever since. There were times when I saw you overdosed on pills and wished you would die." Three days later he told me he hated our older daughter because she reminded him of me. With that, he was out. I asked him to leave that night and I filed for a divorce the following Monday.

During the divorce, I started working as a representative for a pharmaceutical company, selling drugs and being trained that there's always something you can take for anything. There was a part of my mind that said if a doctor wrote it out, that meant it was innocent and harmless, and I just didn't connect prescription drugs with drug taking, per se, even when I stole them from a doctor's office, which I did a lot.

I started drinking again after the divorce and continued doing speed periodically. I was constantly being addicted, detoxed and readdicted. I used speed because I was addicted to food and, because the speed kept me from sleeping at night, I used Valium on a daily basis. It's like peeling onions—layers and layers of addictions. People think, well, I can take lots and lots of Valium for a month or two and not get into trouble. But it's not like that, because Valium stores up in your brain and vital organs.

"I was taking so much, I'd forget what I took."

I didn't know that I was addicted to Valium until I went on a Thanksgiving trip to my brother's in 1978. When we got up there I realized I had forgotten my Valium and started feeling crazy. My body tightened up. I knew that my sister-in-law took Valium so I went on a hunt all over the house and finally found it in her purse and stole it. As soon I took the pill the symptoms went away. That was the first glimpse I had that I might be in trouble.

I moved into a little two-story house with the two girls and I looked at it as a new beginning, but things really started getting bad. It took more and more Valium to anesthetize me. I was losing my memory. I would wake up and feel a lot of disconnection and couldn't remember what day it was. If I had to call home, I had to call information to get my number. I'd constantly lose my keys, my purse. My job was getting a lot more difficult. They were adding real sophisticated drugs that I had to study and pass tests with the FDA in order to sell. I'd be okay if they tested me the following day, but if it was more than twenty-four hours I'd have forgotten everything. I just couldn't retain it.

My relationships were getting really sick. I was drawing abusive, ill men to me, mirroring my own illness. Just about everyone I was attracted to was on something. I had only glimpses of what was happening. It was like looking through fog. For instance, I had always been a real attentive mother. I'd spend a lot of time preparing the kids' meals and those little things. But one day I was sitting in the living room when I realized it had been months since I had fixed the children dinner. That's the kind of little glimpses I got.

Another thing: I always loved clothes and shopping. Then I realized it had been almost a year since I had bought anything because it was too scary to go into a shopping center. I was having trouble with crowds, having lots of anxiety attacks, feeling numbness in my hands and feet. Valium can produce agoraphobic symptoms and that's what was happening to me. It got harder and harder to do my job. Here I am in sales and I'm afraid to go outside and I'm afraid to talk with people. It was a very painful time. I had been back to AA and stopped drinking for a few months, but I was always loaded on pills.

Toward the end, I had no idea what I was taking. I was taking so much, I'd forget what I took. I had discontinued the speed because it made me go immobile, like somebody starched me. I couldn't even talk. So all I took was tranquilizers. And the more I took, the more anxious I'd become.

"I got real clear there was no human power that could help me."

One day I couldn't remember where I had hidden my drugs and I couldn't get in to see any of the doctors I knew. Within twenty- four hours I was in a full anxiety attack. It started with a feeling of impending doom. Then I began to shake and sweat and my teeth chattered. My muscles cramped up and I was terrified.

I found my way down to the clubhouse where all the AA people I knew hung out. I sat among a small group and all they talked about was people they knew who had the dual problem of pills and alcohol. As soon as they brought up pills I tried to change the subject. But halfway through the evening it flashed on me, like somebody picked me up and shook me and said, "My God, you know what's wrong with you? *You're addicted.*"

By this time I was in severe pain. I walked over to a woman who was having dinner and announced, "Jan, I've got to tell you something: I think I'm addicted to Valium." "Why do you think that?" she said. "Because it's been twelve hours since my last pill," I said, "and I think I'm going crazy."

Today if you walked into an AA meeting and said that to somebody, they'd send you straight to a hospital. Five years ago they didn't have a lot of information on pills and she said, "Well, we can't do anything tonight. Just go home, stay put and we'll see what we can do tomorrow."

I was practically near seizure at this point but I got in the car, and drove back to my house screaming. The fear was intense and everything happening in my body was so frightening, I was just walking through hell. I couldn't sleep. My mind was racing back in my life, digging up details, my body was twitching and cramping up. I called a close friend who drove over to spend the night with me. Every hour she woke up to see if I was still breathing.

In the morning we called my mother to come take care of the kids. We called another person in AA who said, "Gee, I think if you put her in a Jacuzzi and she jogged for a few days she'd be okay." Finally we got to the right person who said, "Get this woman to a treatment center. Do not pass go. Take her to Dr. Carr who has some experience with Valium." I called the woman I had spoken to at the clubhouse the night before. She said, "You have to go to an AA meeting before you go to a hospital." I could have fallen over dead, but I went to the meeting. I was an awful thing to see, shaking, crying, my teeth chattering and my body in a lot of pain. After the meeting, they took me to the hospital.

The first thing they said when I got there was, "My God, why did she wait? People like her have seizures and die." They medicated me a bit to give my body a rest before they brought me down. Five years ago they brought people down very hard. Today they bring them down as soft as they can. Addicts may go emotionally nuts but they don't have to go through the physical pain I went through.

Initially, they gave me some medication but once they started the process I didn't sit, sleep, or lay down for days. I walked the floor just like an animal, up and down the hall, in and out of my little room. My mind was racing, my body was cramped up, I cried for days. One night a heroin addict who was walking up and down there with me said, "My God, what is that stuff you're on? I've never seen anything like this." "It's Valium," I told him. He said, "God, I won't ever touch that stuff!" There was another woman in there for Valium, one year younger than me, who died. She was thirty-six years old and her heart just couldn't take it.

I was in a rage of crying with a lot of stuff coming up out of the past. All I could think of were all the bad things, how I'd been in cracker factories and woken up in rubber rooms, how my whole life has been about abuse, how as a child love to me meant pain. For seven days I was just like a wounded animal. I was in the grip of negative thoughts I had no power to stop. And this was a turning point for me. I got real clear that there was no human power that could help me. This was where, for the very first time, I hit my knees and reached out in prayer. I asked God to help me, to come into my heart and let me know what I needed to do and reveal to me what I needed to know—about my father, about my life, and myself. It took seven days to get to that first surrender.

"I started to surrender and pray and the pain went away."

The first point of surrender was when I stopped dwelling on the bad and started looking at some of the good. I looked at the fact that my children were healthy and I was still alive. I relived the time I actually gave birth to my son when they put him in my arms and I looked at him for the first time. It was at this point that all the pain stopped. All the crampings stopped. I felt like God had put his hands around me. It was a real miracle and I saw it as such. As soon as I started looking at the good, praying and asking God to help me and to deliver me from all this, all the really bad stuff stopped. And the miracle was, I was able to go back to my room and sit on my bed, without any pain, for the first time in seven days.

The next day, my friend came to see me and as soon as she walked into the room she knew something had happened. First of all I was sitting fairly quiet. "Did you sleep last night?" she asked. I said, "No, I didn't sleep but I could lay in my bed." I talked to her about the night before. "You know, Judy" I said, "there might be something to this God stuff. I started to surrender and pray, and the pain went away."

Then I talked about my father, calling him "my dad," and with those two words my body got so stiff I practically flew off the bed and I began screaming. All the rage and hate and anger that I had carried from the incest and used the Valium to anesthetize—now that all the drugs were gone there was nothing to hold it down. It was like a pressure cooker. All the crying of the past days was the bubbling of the rage. And so with "my dad" I screamed out years, years of rage, like an exorcism.

Initially they came in to shoot me up, but I wouldn't let them touch me. I didn't understand what was happening but I knew it was something significant and I screamed this stuff up for a long time. It was as though my father was in the room. I forgave him. And when I forgave him, I forgave me. It was the most wonderful process: a spiritual healing.

The trouble with incest victims is, they always feel they're responsible and at fault. But when I was able to let my dad off the hook, I let me off the hook and the most amazing thing happened. Until this point I never let anyone see too much of me. I hid my face behind a lot of fake hair. I lived in wigs. You could see me within a week's time and I would have three or four very different looks. Some days it would be long hair, some days short hair, different makeup, different styles. I became all these people and distanced myself by being incognito. That day I looked at myself in the mirror and for the first time I felt connected to myself.

That same day, I had some flowers sent to me. They came in a great big basket and each flower was perfect. There was not a brown mark on anything. I took that as a message that I was returned to that perfection. God was telling me, "This is how you are." And I started opening up.

"In the vision I was wearing a white suit, a black blouse . . ."

My counselors at the treatment center came and said, "If you want what we have, you're going to have to quit your job and stop selling drugs." I was making fifty thousand dollars a year, more than most men I knew. I had a new car in my driveway every two years. So I just panicked. I thought, "What am I going to do? How am I going to support these children?" "Well," they said, "you've been doing okay with surrender so far. Why don't you just turn this one over to God?" And before I went to bed that night I got on my knees and asked God to give me the willingness to do what I had to do and resign from the job. And then I asked Him to reveal to me what He wanted me to do in life. I was real open to His directions, and then I had a vision.

In the vision I was wearing a white suit, a black blouse and standing up at a podium with hundreds of people in front of me. I had no idea what that meant and I was afraid to tell anyone about it, so I just kept it to myself. The following day I called my company and resigned. I went from fifty thousand dollars a year to six hundred dollars a month disability.

And then they came and said, "Thirty days here is not going to do the trick. You're going to have to go to some long-term recovery house." I said, "I can't go because of the kids." And they said, "Why don't you pray about it and turn this one over to God, too?" I said, "God's going to have to go some on this, because I don't have any family living in town."

The next day my brother and sister-in-law called and said, "We're thinking of moving to your neck of the woods. Can we stay at your place for the summer so we get a chance to look at jobs and housing?" "As a matter of fact," I said, "they're trying to ship me out of here for the summer. Can the kids stay with you?" And they said, "Sure, we'd love it." God's perfection!

So they shipped me off to a place called Placel in St. Louis. I did a lot of praying, studying and developing myself spiritually with meditation. I had this sense while I was there that I was just buying time and letting everything heal. I had no idea what I was going to do when I got back home.

Placel was an intermediate house. After about three months, I went back home to a halfway house, where I had more freedom. I was beginning to get my memory back, but I was still very disconnected and didn't feel a lot. I'd get lost and panicky in shopping centers. I'd forget where I was so I needed to go out with women who were a little further along than I was. I was still having anxiety attacks and I still couldn't drive.

I was about five months clean and sober when I started going home. I went home gradually, at first only on weekends. I was still disconnected, but I began to drive, not freeways but little access streets.

I started volunteering at a hospital, talking to the patients who were coming off pills. My thinking processes and reaction time were very slow at first, but they began coming back. My feelings and my memory slowly returned, too, and I began to be interested in having a relationship with a man again.

From the moment I forgave my father I never again attracted an abusive man. From that point on, all the men who came into my life were gentle, loving, caring men. I was about a year and a half sober when I got in a relationship with a real soft, gentle man. He wasn't the love of my life but it was real warm and I learned to be friends. We quit smoking together and it was a healthy relationship.

Then I met Jason, a wonderful, compassionate man. We've been married for a year now and he's my best friend. And I have a relationship today with my father that is built on forgiveness and love, and a relationship with my kids that is just incredibly close and loving. And it was all through a spiritual program and surrender after surrender after surrender. For a woman who has gone through incest and twenty years with an abusive husband to come out the other end in this kind of recovery, it's nothing less than a miracle.

One day the hospital called me and asked me to come to work for them. I didn't have any degree in counseling and, other than volunteering, I had no experience working in the field. But they brought me in and I started their outpatient program. One day they said, "We'd like you to do Outreach. It's public speaking and educating the community." "No," I said, "I don't want to do that." But the next day and I went back and accepted.

The first talk I gave was at a high school where I stood at a podium before three hundred parents. I looked out and it was *deja vu*. I looked down and I had on the white suit and the black blouse. The scene was exactly the way I had dreamed it. Exactly.

Now I have a whole staff of people and a reputation as a public speaker. And monetarily I've gone from five dollars an hour to off the charts. But I think the greatest thing has been learning how to receive love. I've learned about intimacy and allowing a man in to get close to me. In my childhood, my father beat the sh— out of me and when he finished he'd say, "I do that because I love you." So I associated love with pain. And for me to have a relationship today that's based on love without pain is a real miracle.

So the hope is with surrender. I really believe that if people go through this kind of pain you have no choice but to let go. And what happens is—it's in the power of letting go and that surrender that you get the power back. And that's when major changes occur, that's where you move mountains. It's been proven over and over that if I was willing to get out of my own way great things would happen to me, and they have.

4

Barbiturates and Antidepressants Laura's Story

From Sleep to Suicide

Barbiturates were introduced in 1903, under the trade name Veronal. By the 1930s, Americans were consuming one billion grains a year.[1] In the forties the American Medical Association, alarmed by the widespread abuse of barbiturates, published an article entitled "1,250,000,000 Doses a Year." By 1969, *ten billion* doses a year were being produced. A survey at one college indicated that a quarter of the students had used them.[2] Only a few years ago, barbiturates accounted for three-fourths of all drug deaths.[3] Three hundred tons of barbiturates are currently manufactured every year in this country, half of which find their way into the illicit drug market.[4]

Despite a decline in barbiturate use over the past decade, they are still abused on a vast scale, and they are still predominantly a woman's drug.[5] In a 1982 NIDA study listing the twelve most abused prescription drugs, three were barbiturates (Luminal, Seconal, and Tuinal) and two were barbiturate-like compounds (Placidyl and Doriden).[6] In 1984, eight thousand emergency room visits by women were associated with their use and they were the third most frequently cited class of drugs in female suicides.[7]

The barbiturates have a particularly vicious nature. They are used to treat anxiety, but taken in the presence of mental stress, they can cause delirium.[8] They are used as sleeping aids, but they prevent the very kind of sleep that is essential to feeling well-rested.[9] And while tolerance to their effects develops quickly, little tolerance develops to their lethal dose level. A long-time user of barbiturates is as prone to crossing the fatal line as a newcomer.[10]

The barbiturates, like all sedatives, do one thing superbly well: they get the user drunk. Their effect on moving, thinking, and personality are practically indistinguishable from alcohol's.[11] A woman on a barbiturate initially feels a reduction of guilt and anxiety. This mood alteration—called disinhibition euphoria—changes to increased emotional instability, loss of coordination, unsteadiness in walking, slurred speech and difficulty in thinking clearly.[12] In the "morning after" hangover, barbiturates are frequently used to treat the very symptoms they have caused.

The barbiturate-like compounds, such as Doriden and Placidyl, were developed as safer alternative drugs, but they have no real advantages over the barbiturates, and in fact have several disadvantages. Because the range between Doriden's therapeutic dose and lethal dose is narrow, an overdose is extremely difficult to reverse and frequently results in death.[13,14] And, because Doriden remains in the stomach even longer than the barbiturates, it can be reabsorbed and produce coma *after* the user appears to have recovered from an overdose.[15]

Placidyl is marketed as a safe barbiturate substitute, but its manufacturer admits that it "has the potential for the development of psychological and physical dependence" and that "instances of severe withdrawal symptoms, including convulsions are . . . clinically similar to those seen with barbiturates."[16] Placidyl is also highly fat soluble, which means it stays in a woman's body a long time.[17]

Any of these drugs taken during pregnancy can lead to withdrawal symptoms in the newborn baby, including restlessness, sleeplessness, persistent high-pitched cry, and occasional convulsions. These symptoms can be more severe than those experienced in narcotic withdrawal, and they frequently do not appear until several days after birth, and recur until the child is six months old.[18]

Barbiturates and barbiturate-like drugs resemble alcohol in withdrawal as well as in intoxication, and kicking them can be a difficult experience, especially if high doses have been taken for a long time. At first a woman withdrawing from barbiturates can appear to be sobering up. Then weakness, anxiety, and depression set in, followed by the shakes. At its worst, barbiturate withdrawal includes delirium tremens, a life-threatening syndrome of delusions, hallucinations, profuse sweating and high fever.[19] Sudden withdrawal from the barbiturates carries a risk of brain seizure and death. For these reasons, barbiturate abusers are cautioned not to attempt any withdrawal on their own, but to seek responsible professional help, preferably in an inpatient treatment center setting.

The woman setting out on the road to sedative-free living needs to understand that the physical and psychological pain she may experience can no longer be fixed by her pills, but is the inevitable by-product of the drugs themselves. She needs to understand that her pain, self-doubt, and fears are normal and temporary. With the proper care and support, particularly from those women who have themselves overcome barbiturate dependency, these drugs can be kicked for good.

In the story that follows, barbiturates play a major role, but Laura also frequently talks about another class of drugs: the tricyclic antidepressants. These antidepressants include Amitril, Elavil, Amitriptyline, Sinequan, Tofranil, and others. The progression from barbiturates to antidepressants is not uncommon.

The tricyclic antidepressants are among the newest drugs in a doctor's pharmacopia. Not surprisingly, they are touted as safe, nonaddictive drugs with low abuse potential. In the AMA's drug abuse guide for the primary care physician, they are glaringly ignored. Yet they are a factor in more female drug suicides than *any* class of drugs.[20]

The tricyclics are prescribed as antidepressants and sedatives. They alter mood, lift worries, improve alertness and sleep and induce a sense of well-being.[21] They clearly have an effect, but are they necessary?

A recent major study by the National Institute of Mental Health found that tricyclic antidepressants are no more effective for depression than brief psychotherapy.[22]

The tricyclic antidepressents are a particular scourge to older women. Three times as many women over sixty-five as men use sedatives and antidepressants.[23] The side effects of these drugs among the elderly include dry mouth, constipation, blurred vision, and urinary problems. The half-life of these drugs is twice as long in elderly women as in younger women, so their effects persist that much longer.[24] They can lower blood pressure to the point of causing dizziness when the user stands up, which can lead to falls and broken bones.[25] Another set of effects they commonly produce is a state of confusion, short-term memory impairment, hallucinations, and disorientation—symptoms that sound remarkably similar to senility. In fact, some researchers are concluding that many cases of presumed senility are really reactions to overmedicating with antidepressants.

As Laura's story illustrates, the tricyclics are sometimes used to treat the depression that accompanies alcoholism. If a woman resumes heavy drinking while under tricyclic medication, the effect can lead to coma and death.[26] Because the popularity of the tricyclic antidepressants continues to grow, they are sometimes called the Valium of the nineties. We can expect to hear more stories of their abuse.

In Laura's story we meet a drug-dependent woman who outwardly seemed to be living an almost stereotypically American life—successful husband, children, and a house with a white picket fence. But behind that fence, a lot more besides drug abuse was going on. Laura was also a battered and raped wife.

*   *   *

Laura's Story

*Laura is an amiable, outgoing woman. With her long
hair and petite figure, it is hard to believe she is the
mother of two fully grown children. We interviewed her
at her home. She looked comfortable in slacks and tee
shirt. She made us feel comfortable, too.*

I was born and raised in Detroit in a lower middle-class family—the
working-hard class. My father was a dry alcoholic. I don't remember
him ever drinking. My mother was raised in the Depression. She lost
her father real young and lived in an orphanage. When she married
my father, who was nine years older than her, she never called him
by his first name. She always called him Daddy. She catered to my
father's two children from his first marriage, a boy and a girl, who
were ten and twelve years older than me, so my sister and I were
forgotten.

Throughout my childhood, my mother took lots of pills: thyroid
pills, nerve pills, all that stuff. I didn't realize until recently how
much was there for me to imitate, but from the time I was seven or
eight, I used to steal the bottle of orange-flavored baby aspirin and
eat them all. I was always an aspirin freak. I never saw it like that. I
just always took them.

I went to a very wealthy parish Catholic school where we were
the charity case and I was always reminded of that, by my mother
and by the nuns. My mother put me in dresses that were too long
because they were my older sister's and I had to grow into them. It
was real humiliating. She never made an effort to make my sister
and me look decent. My half-sister and brother never had to dress
funny. They always looked fine.

"I thought they were going to kill me."

By the time I was in fourth grade, I had nephritis, a kidney disease,
but I never knew I had it. My parents never told me I was sick. On
the night of my confirmation my mom said, "We're going out for a

ride. We'll come back in a second." We drove to the hospital and they all waited in the car while my mom took me upstairs and dumped me. It was horrible. I thought they did it because I was a bad girl—because I whined and cried too much, or spilled my milk, or wouldn't eat my vegetables. I said, "Aren't I going to get a party?" "Well, no," she said, "you have to stay here." She left me with the words, "I'll see you in the morning." The next morning my mom didn't make it.

The nurses came and took me downstairs to the operating room. They strapped me down, first my arms, then my legs—because they were going to do all this internal stuff. I was raised on "naughty" and "dirty" and "nasty" and all this no-no stuff about the body. They laid me down and strapped my legs apart. I wanted to die. I thought they were going to kill me because I had been such a bad girl.

"I realized it was fun to get away."

The first time I ever took pills was after we moved to California, when I was fifteen. I was in high school. I was real unhappy and miserable. I didn't fit in. I bought the over-the-counter drug that puts you to sleep, I think it was Sleep-eze. So I took these pills and that's when I realized it was fun to get away.

I got married to my first husband, Frank, right out of high school and worked at a job for just over a year. But I had to quit because of high blood pressure. My doctor gave me a prescription for some pills. He said I couldn't drink while I was taking these pills, but we were newly married and all we did was party.

Very quickly I learned that you really *could* drink and take these pills. And it was *that much better* if you drank and took these pills.

After about a year, I had just found out I was pregnant when my husband got drafted and sent to Vietnam. "God," I prayed, "don't make me move home to my mother. Anything but that!" But I had to and it was horrible. I was despondent the whole time.

"I fell madly in love with Seconal."

I had just turned twenty-one when my daughter was born. I was having nightmares about my husband getting killed in the war. I existed for the last year as this fat, depressed woman whose husband was gone. I didn't know what to do with the baby. Then there was the stress of the war, watching it on the news all the time. Throughout this time, I was drinking and taking aspirins.

I went to the doctor and told him about the nightmares, that I was paranoid and nervous and just beside myself. So he put me on Meprobamate, Miltown. They were some of the strongest pills I ever took and I adored them.

It was time for my husband to get a pass for some R and R in Hawaii in July. A girlfriend and I went to buy my airline ticket. On the way to the airport, she said, "Look I've got these reds we ought to try." I said, "Great." So we stopped at a gas station, took a Seconal each and got so screwed up that by the time we reached the airport, all we could do was park. We looked at each other and drove straight home and I crashed.

I fell madly in love with Seconal. That's what I wanted to feel the rest of my life. Out. Gone. No feelings, nothing. Just numb. I was hooked on them. If I had had a barrel of them I would have taken them all.

I finally got to Hawaii with my baby and we stayed for a couple of months. I drank a lot over there. When we came back in September, I had bad menstrual cramps. I always had a lot of problems with that part of my life. I used to spend weeks in bed, but now I had my baby and I couldn't do that.

So the doctor prescribed a darling little green pill that looked like green aspirin. I'd alternate between them and my barbs. My doctor told me to take two to four of the green pills, but why take two when you can take four? I didn't think they were that strong, but all I would do when I took them was drink coffee, smoke and get a lot done. Then a few days later I'd come crashing down, kind of recover and go back on downers. Eventually I did both at the same time.

At a certain point I became aware that those little green pills were speed. But then, they weren't really. They were medication. It was always medication. And I needed them. I wasn't going to take anything just for fun! Never, in all the years I took drugs, was I on *drugs*. It was always *nerve pills*. It was always *medicine*. I would have been terribly offended had anyone called it anything else.

Then my husband was wounded.

"I just sat there hating him."

When Frank was sent home, he was practically dead. His head had been damaged by mortar, and they had to operate and remove a lot of his brain. I went to the hospital every day in the morning and sat and nursed him all day. He was half-paralyzed. I had this baby and my mother and now this a—hole gets blown up and I'm thinking, "This is great. Thanks a lot!" So I just sat there hating him.

Most of the time he was out of it, close to a coma. But when he rallied he was real ugly and mean. He would kick food on me. In the hospital, I made friends with this kid in the pharmacy who said, "Look, you're really uptight. I'll get you something from the pharmacy." So it got to be that every few days this guy used to go and scoop up an envelope of darling little Libriums and hand them to me.

Here I am in the hospital hating my husband and you can't drink while you're there, so I'd go into the bathroom and pop pills. Then I didn't give a sh—. Go ahead and be a creep to me.

"I realized I was in trouble."

I took these pills all day long. I was still taking Miltown in the morning to get out the door, and drinking at night. I knew that the pills were so powerful, I could kill myself with them. So I would cut them in half, take half a pill and drink.

Then I got real crazy. When I tried to drive my car off a cliff, I realized I was in trouble. My gynecologist, who was the only person I confided in, said, "You need a psychiatrist." The psychiatrist put me in a hospital. So here we go.

The hospitalization was great. They gave me whatever: Melaril, Elavil, Nembutal, Librium, and Thorazine. God, Thorazine. Doing the Thorazine shuffle. You can't do anything else. You can't lift your legs. You can only shuffle through. I liked it though. I never wanted to move fast anyway. The mellower the better.

I would get a prescription and tell the doctor about the side effects and he would give me something new. I kept the other pills and learned that was a great way to accumulate lots of stash. I would take pills for four or five days, call him and say, "They make me feel funny," and he would say, "Fine, let's find something else." Meanwhile, I developed symptoms of arthritis, so I'm going to another doctor who was also prescribing medications, double-teaming them both.

"I could take the speed and do a hell of a job."

I was raking in this pile of pills and I used to hide them. I always had the ones I really cared for in my purse. I never wanted to be away from them. I hid the others under the bed, in drawers, in the trunk of my car.

The pills were the closest part of my identity. Booze was definitely secondary. But through it all, I made it look good by drinking. I covered up the pills with alcohol.

My life was shattered. I had a husband who was not going to come around. No one told me things like this could happen to you in real life! . . . I ended up getting a divorce from Frank.

By this time I am taking so many pills and I'm back to work for the first time in a long time. Now, if I had cramps, they said, "Oh, go to the medical department, they'll give you something for it." When I went there I found out that "something" was the little green speed pills. I thought, "Terrific." I was so hung over when I got to work, I could take the speed and do a hell of a job. Then I'd go to another department and say, "Hey, can I borrow yours because I don't have enough time to go over there?" So I was collecting from two departments. And that's how I got through work. I took the speed and did a lot of work. About once every two weeks I did all my work and then I'd kind of f— off in the meantime.

Now I'm at the point that I don't know whether I'm coming or going from the pills because I'm going up and coming down at the same time. I ended up having another nervous breakdown.

"I was carted off by the police."

By the time I went into the hospital again, I had been in a blackout for about two weeks. I don't remember anything that happened. I stayed in for two months for pill addiction.

The hospital wouldn't give me any pills. Not birth control pills, not aspirin, not anything. I'd watch the other patients going for pill calls three or four times a day and I just had to sit there.

I didn't want to get off pills, and yet I was scared. It was still medication, not using. I "had" to take them.

A heroin addict was in there with me and a guy who got bummed out from an LSD trip. The heroin addict had a great time, because they nursed him down. They were giving all this other medication to the LSD guy. But I was going crazy.

I would sit down at the table and be fine. Then all of sudden, I felt, these people are moving too much, I have to get out of here. I ran to my room, was terrified of being alone and ran back.

Or if I were in my car, I'd think, they're moving too fast, and I'd pull off on the side of the freeway. I was carted off by the police a couple of times because I just wanted everyone to stop. I had to have my car picked up from various places.

I panicked at work. I'd say, "I just have to go outside." Then I'd panic outside and go back in. I called my sister at her job and told her I had to get away from there, to come and pick me up. She left her job and came to get me. She drove an hour to take me to her house. By the time she got back to *her* office, I had called someone at *my* office to come and get me. This happened on both sides of the hospital experience.

I was in the hospital for about three months, and no one ever mentioned I couldn't have alcohol. So when they let me go home on weekends to see my daughter, I picked up a bottle on the way, was drunk all weekend and checked myself back in on Monday. They never said anything about the way alcohol and pills were related.

"Raising five children was really bizarre."

When I got out, the doctor said, "You *do* need something." He gave me a prescription for Valium. That was the first time I ever had Valium.

I was losing my job. That's when I decided to marry Bob. He was an engineer and had a house in La Jolla. I married him for the security. Plus he had a terrific stash of marijuana. He and his family had drugs. But Bob was just a real cold man who needed somebody to babysit his three kids.

After we got married, the doctor became strict about my pills and gave them to my husband. Bob got up in the morning, went to the safe and poured out three or four Valiums for the day and handed them to me. I thought, "Hey, buster, number one, who wants four pills, and number two, I hate you." Eventually, I broke the safe with a crowbar and got my stash back and hid it.

When I had Valium, I started gaining weight again. After my second baby, I never completely lost the extra weight. I told my shrink I wanted diet pills, and he said, "I don't think that's a good idea." I said, "Fine, I'll get them off the street." He said, "Okay, I'll give them to you." He gave me a real powerful diet pill.

I also had two stepsons who were hyperkinetic. They had to see a shrink once a month who gave them each a prescription for a nice tall bottle of speed, Ritalin, that they had to take at school. But I changed the dosage so I could keep one bottle for me. Then eventually I decided they should really be off Ritalin because it was addictive. I took them to their appointment and got the prescription, but I kept it all.

I was still drinking a lot and taking barbs. I *never* stopped taking barbs. I don't care how much speed I took, I took barbs because that kept my feelings off as much as possible. That was the main point for me. To not feel anything. Maybe because as a child I was not allowed to feel. I was not allowed to act the way I felt. I was always told, "Knock it off." I was always told to stop how I was feeling. So I would change the outside, but the inside stayed the same. Which is why I grew up so confused about the way I felt. The exterior was not the same as the interior, which is why I was convinced of what a rotten, sick, crazy person I was. I was always being told to act different than I was.

Now, married to Bob it was the same thing all over again. He would go off to work and there I'd be with five children: three of his, one of mine and one of ours. He would go off to work oblivious to the fact that raising five children was really bizarre.

I sat around with all my emotions hanging out talking about the kids driving me crazy and he would say, "Well, if you just did this or that, it would be fine." He totally did not hear me.

I was now seeing my shrink once a week and still getting pills from him. And having side effect upon side effect. Valium made me slur. Thorazine made me shuffle. But even with all the pills I was taking, I was always on the verge of explosion with the kids.

I wanted my house tidy all the time. If I smoked a cigarette, I got up and washed the ashtray out. I sat and watched the kids playing and if I saw a piece of lint, I would pick it up. That was my whole life: fluffing, folding, sandwich making, producing meals. And I hated it.

"I was black and blue from this man."

Right from the beginning of those five years of our marriage, I think it was in the second week, he slapped me. Occasionally he beat me up. One time he dragged me out on the porch and banged my head on the cement, telling me how good it felt to be doing this to me.

At one point we both went to the shrink who said it was time for group—you know, marriage counseling. I remember sitting there, talking to my husband, talking about his beating me up, and he was sitting there saying, "I may have slapped her, I never beat her up." I was black and blue. Black and blue from this man.

Well: I felt it was my fault. Maybe I was making a mountain out of a molehill. After all, I'm just the wife. I am a woman who is supposed to make the beds and keep the house running and he's the breadwinner. And basically how I felt is ". . . and I'm the nothing." Which led me to take more pills.

We bought a new house. He let me pick it out. It was *the* house. You'd drive up Wisteria Drive in beautiful Point Loma and see two Cape Cod houses and five little darling children. The grass is green, there are kittycats, the aroma coming out of the kitchen. And the man of the house—he beats me up. And I'm miserable. And who cares? That's what happens in America all the time.

I could look out the window at the Mormon family across the street. The woman was my age with six or seven babies. She'd be mowing the lawn or baking bread with kids on her shoulders screaming and she was smiling. I just wanted to die.

"So I started hiding in my house."

Once, after I had gotten beaten up, Bob was going to take his children away for Easter vacation and I decided I was going to commit suicide and was taking *my* children with me. I had saved all these pills and I was going to put them in the hot chocolate. I had these great suicide notes. I think I just got too screwed up to get it done.

I was seeing my shrink and taking so many pills that I didn't know what I was doing. I got up in the morning and I drank as well. The drinking was a real good cover. You would get drunk, too, if you took as many pills as I did. It was a lot better to let people think I was an alcoholic than for anyone to take my pills. Taking my pills was like taking my arms.

I had had blackouts on pills years and years ago but now my blackouts were constant, every day, all the time. I never remembered beyond dinner with the kids. I couldn't remember how they got put to bed, or bathing them or anything. When I woke up the next morning, I was the first one down the stairs and I'd find my car keys in the door and the door open and the car in a different place.

I tried to keep track of how many pills I took by marking them on the calendar, but I never knew what all those marks meant. Does that mean that I've taken enough for today? I probably was just taking them every ten or fifteen minutes all day, all the time, because I was going through them like they were water. I had to swallow pills because I knew they would make it okay. They just made it all *bearable*, and that's all it ever was.

I was taking everything the doctors would give me: Ritalin, Valium, Nembutal, Seconal, Miltown, Stellazine. I never liked Stellazine. They never seemed to do much. So I took a lot of them, like fillers, like oatmeal in your meatloaf. I knew people who died taking less than half of what I took and I never even got my stomach pumped. I went into blackouts for weeks on end but I never . . . I think that God just had plans for me and that's the way it was.

I fantasized burning my house to the ground all the time. I just wanted to destroy everything. I felt like I was in this cage and all I did all day long, for years, was pace. Around and around. *Just like a caged animal.* I'd get in my rocking chair and I'd rock and I'd rock. That was soothing.

I was so paranoid. Whenever my family got together I *knew* they were plotting to put me away. So I started hiding in my house. I would run and hide in the corner, afraid that they would see me.

Finally, I had a brother-in-law who'd gone to AA and I went and saw him get an anniversary cake and something happened.

"So my husband came home one night and raped me."

I told my psychiatrist, "I think that I might be an alcoholic." He asked me why and I don't remember what I said but I told him, "I think I'm going to go to an AA meeting."

I went to an AA meeting. People said, "Come back." I didn't have to be at home with this man I hated and all these children. I had quit being able to do any more laundry, any more cooking. I was done. My husband used to say to me, "If you don't go to a meeting tonight, I'll let you smoke a joint." I asked him why he didn't want me to go to AA and he said, "I'm afraid if you go to AA you'll leave me."

Which is exactly what happened. One night I packed my suitcase. I took a vial of pills, a fifth of booze, a bag of ice, my yellow suicide tablets and cigarettes to a motel to kill myself.

But again I got too screwed to do anything, so I called a man in AA and asked him to come and talk to me. He came and put me in a car and drove me around. But I ran away from him because, when he got out to pump gas, I *knew* he actually got out to call my husband to get the paddywagon from the looney bin. I hid in the bushes until dark.

I was sure they were going to lock me up and that I would be crazy all my life because I was bad. I was a bad mother. I was a bad wife. I was a bad daughter. I was just bad. Bad, bad, bad.

I went back to my husband, kept going to meetings, and actually stopped drinking. But I still couldn't give up pills. Pill addicts have a lot harder time getting clean than alcoholics. Because our brain is different. We're so squirrely. That's what it's like, all these squirrels running around in your head. My brain itched. It was horrible.

I had made friends in AA with a man named Norm. We were never lovers, but my husband found a note that Norm had written me and assumed we were having an affair. So my husband came home one night and raped me.

I thought, "That, f—er, is it!" I went downstairs and lay in bed with a fishing knife. I was going to stab him. If he opens that door, he's a dead man. I watched the doorknob all night long. As soon as it was daylight, I called my parents and said, "I'm leaving him, can I come there?" I took my two children.

"I want to come out clean."

Somewhere along the line in the AA meetings I was going to, somebody said I had to stop taking the pills. I thought, "I *am* off pills."

But every night, I came home from the meeting and took these pills called Equanil, a mood elevator and some kind of mild tranquilizer that a doctor had given me for "manic depression." I automatically reached over my sink for my pills and I never even *counted* them as pills. And of course I always had my Seconals and Nembutals just in case I needed something stronger.

People would say, "God, I'm having trouble sleeping nights," and I'd think, "God, I slept fine when I was newly sober. . . ."

But when I got off my little pills, then the party was over.

That was when I had been ten months without alcohol. I had to have a hysterectomy. I thought, "Now is the time!" I was hooked on AA, I was hooked on the people, on the fact that they were saying, You're okay.

I went to my gynecologist and we made this deal. "When I come out of the hospital, I want to come out clean. I want to stop *everything.*"

He was all for the idea because he had been trying to get me to stop for some time. So when I had the operation I said that three days into recovery, I wanted no more pills.

He talked to my anesthesiologist about it. He made it very clear to everybody that this is what we were going to do. They could give me barbiturates and whatever else they thought I needed while I was there, but once I left, I wouldn't take anything ever again.

I had *fifty* visitors when I was in the hospital. I kept a log of all the people because I was so jazzed that people liked me. That gave me the strength to get clean.

"But I knew I had to go through with it."

I wasn't out of the hospital more than one day when I got violently ill. There was no sleeping, there was no sitting still. You talk about pacing! I felt like my elbows went the wrong way. My skin was on wrong. It was a horrible withdrawal. But I knew I had to go through with it and I had great people help me get through it.

I was such a basket case when I got clean that I didn't know how to do anything. I had to be told what to do, from cleaning the house to raising my kids. That's how I developed my relationship to a higher power. I was terrified of going to the market and terrified of the laundromat. The choices were just overwhelming to me. So I would go to the store and, because of people in AA, I'd say things like, "Okay, God, you decide which cereal and I'll get it."

I trusted that God was giving me the right stuff. That's how God proved himself to me, all these little silly things like surviving a day without burning the kids' tomato soup. I even couldn't cook anymore! But I kept trying. And I talked to women on the phone every day at five o'clock, because that was my roughest time, when I felt I was coming apart over the little things. You know, "Don't spill the milk!"

"All I ever wanted was to be okay."

I met a man, Jeff, who was also a recovering alcoholic and drug addict and we started living together. Everything was going along fine. Then after being sober for two years, I took my first part-time job at a school where I had to lift heavy loads of dishes and I tore a rib. Every breath I took hurt. I went to a doctor who said, "We're going to give you Valium." I said, "I can't have Valium. I'm a drug addict. Don't you have anything else?" So he gave me a tape to wrap around me, and a prescription for Valium. I thought, "You f—ing a—hole," and I tore it up on the way home. I am an addict and this guy is just shoving it at me.

That happened to me on many occasions in my sobriety. At one hospital, when I had the flu, they said, "You take this cough medicine," filled with alcohol and something else, and I reminded them, "But I'm a drug addict." And they said, "Yes, fine, but you just take these." And I'd think, "Why do I come here?" So now I don't go to doctors. I just get well.

But my rib really *did* hurt, so I made the decision, with Jeff's help, that I *would* take some Valium. So, he got four Valium and I took them that night because I needed sleep so bad. It was so painful.

I took the pill and slept. Jeff said I got up in the middle of the night and he gave me another one. In the morning, after sleeping real well, he said to me, "Do you want anything?" and I said, "Yeah, get me some more pills."

I heard myself and thought, "Oh my God, here we go." The change was so glaring. I felt a wall come slamming down between me and God and it was dark. That's what drugs did to me.

I had based a decision to take pills on a physical problem, forgetting that emotionally and mentally I am an addict and it just triggered all that stinking thinking crappy self-destructive stuff that just lies there waiting. It'll wait forever.

I looked back at my life and thought how awful it felt to be me. All I ever wanted was to be okay. Let me just be acceptable. Let me be a member of the human race. I don't want to be famous or anything. Just let someone say it's okay for me to be here, and feel it. God is in my life. One Valium and God would be out. I never took another pill.

"When a woman gets self-worth . . ."

I've been sober and clean nine and a half years, but I still look at pills. When people have a pill bottle they can't get open, I say, "Give it here, I can open anything." Someone gets a prescription and I say, "Let me look at them." I ask people, "What are Quaaludes like?" I never got to take Quaaludes.

Nothing in the world makes me feel better than knowing I don't use. Nothing. Because I know that it is only *that* that lets me wrestle and get rid of those horrible feelings I had as a kid. I never felt good about myself in my life until I got clean. Now I really feel, in the last five years especially, that I've been purified. I feel that anything is possible in my life. I feel so good about myself.

It's been quite a process, and it was the hard way but, boy, I'm really free. That much I know. I'm the one who's free.

I also live a real simple life, you know? I just don't care about all that madness. Every once in a while I get out into it and a little bit goes a long way and I think to myself, "Uh oh." I like being real mellow with myself. I hear the birds when they're singing out there and no one else does. But I do, I know they're singing, and it's worth singing about.

I can look myself in the eye. My elbows are where they belong. There's not this huge knot in my stomach. I'm really free.

I never never never never never never never want to get near that misery. I mean, when a woman gets self-worth, self-respect, you just don't easily give that over at all. That's what it's like to look in the mirror and say, "You know, you really are somebody, kiddo."

5

Diet Pills
Diana's Story

The Costs of Slimness

In *Fat Is a Feminist Issue*, psychotherapist Susie Orbach writes, "Success, beauty, wealth, love, sexuality and happiness are promoted [to women] as attached to and depending on slimness . . . . Selling body insecurity to women . . . is a vicious phenomenon."[1] Selling diet pills to women is a vicious phenomenon with a very lucrative underside. In 1981 Americans spent more than 220 million dollars on over-the-counter (OTC) diet pills alone.[2]

Who were the primary consumers? A recent survey of drug use among the nation's high school seniors found that three times as many women seniors as men use diet pills, with half of all female seniors reporting using them in the past year.[3]

All so-called diet pills are really central nervous system stimulants—a class of drugs that includes amphetamines, several drugs that were developed to replace amphetamines, and a wide selection of over-the-counter pills.

Amphetamine, a synthetic compound that mimics adrenalin, the body's own hormone for emergencies, was introduced into American medical practice in 1937. Amphetamine seemed to enhance physical strength while it increased mental capacity; it produced euphoria, elation, and clear-headed alertness; it improved self-confidence. It did all this without any apparent adverse effects. Amphetamine was, in short, another wonder drug.[4]

By the sixties, college students were popping uppers to cram for exams. Truck drivers found they could hit the road for two days without sleeping. And millions of housewives were using them to control their weight and to overcome the boredom and "mild depression" of unfulfilled lives.[5]

Important differences soon developed in the way men and women used amphetamines. Many men were using them for kicks, and they were getting them on the street.[6] Women were using them to cope and were getting their amphetamines from doctors.

Despite research that showed amphetamines were not effective as a diet aid, doctors prescribed diet pills to women as if their patients' lives depended on it. In 1967 thirty-one million amphetamine prescriptions were written for dieting purposes alone, and eighty percent of these prescriptions were for women.[7,8] In 1969, five billion doses of amphetamines were being legally manufactured. Nearly ninety-nine percent were prescribed for weight loss.[9]

By 1970 America was in the midst of an amphetamine epidemic. Nearly eight percent of all medical prescriptions written were for amphetamines.

In that year the Federal Drug Administration finally bowed to strong evidence that amphetamines were not effective in long-term weight-control programs and set limits on their use. Three types of conditions were allowed to be treated by amphetamines: high levels of physical activity in children and adolescents, sleep epilepsy, and short-term weight-control programs for obesity.[10] The FDA thus continued to approve the use of diet pills for weight control even though its experts knew that the effects of amphetamine on weight control were "clinically trivial."[11] Even with these restrictions in place, in 1978 twelve million women were taking stimulants, mostly diet pills.[12]

Since that time, additional restrictions have severely limited amphetamine's legal use, particularly as a weight-control drug. Then, as the national abuse of cocaine and crystal speed grabbed headlines and research money, both public and medical attention passed over amphetamines.

Amphetamines were further pushed from center stage by a string of competing drugs. They were marketed as Preludin, Ritalin, Didrex, Cylert, Sanorex, and a host of other names. These drugs acted like the amphetamines, right down to their adverse effects, but they were said to be nonaddictive and to have only a mild potential for abuse.[13]

The amphetamine epidemic, then, was thought to be finished. A search through the more than one thousand pages of research published by *The International Journal of the Addictions* in 1985 has failed to come up with a single important reference to amphetamines. They are forgotten, but not gone. In 1984 the amphetamines were second only to marijuana as the most commonly abused illicit drugs among high school seniors.[14]

As amphethamines came under increasing controls, drug manufacturers stepped in with diet drugs which looked like amphetamines and promised the same alleged weight reduction benefits but which contained no controlled substances. These over-the-counter drugs were given names like Diadex, Dexatrim and Dietic, names that called to mind the lure of the amphetamines. Their main ingredient is usually Phenylpropanolomine (PPA), a drug originally marketed as a nasal decongestant.[15]

The FDA acknowledges that PPA is hazardous to a significant portion of the population, and the *Journal of the American Medical Association* has reported potentially fatal heart and kidney problems linked to its use.[16] The Drug Abuse Warning Network, which monitors hospitals in twenty-seven metropolitan areas serving only one-third of the U.S. population, reported 746 PPA-caused emergency room visits in 1984, with women outnumbering men four to one.[17]

The up side of all diet pills is the euphoria and sense of boundless energy that they produce. The down side includes the headaches, dizziness, agitation, confusion, fatigue, anxiety, heart palpitations, hallucinations, and depression.[18]

Amphetamine, the most powerful of the diet pills, has the most serious negative effects. Even in low doses, experience of heightened energy can turn to nervousness and jittery feelings.[19] At moderate dose levels the user's outlook typically goes from initial confidence and alertness to apprehension and irritability. Moderate to heavy use may cause the user to get hung up in a simple activity. A woman may spend hours repeating a thought, some words, or a phrase of music.[20] Hallucinations of touch, smell and hearing also occur.[21] The user feels that bugs are crawling under her skin, or that she is losing control and going crazy.[22,23] Higher doses lead to fever, convulsions, paranoia and psychosis. Continued use can lead to cerebral hemorrhaging, and death.[24]

Amphetamines have a high abuse potential because of their rebound effect and the relative ease with which even low doses produce tolerance.[25] The rebound effect is the crash the user feels when the euphoria of the dose wears off.[26] The lethargy and depression of the crash is typically countered by another pill. But because the chronic user easily develops tolerance to a certain dosage of amphetamine, a woman may find herself taking higher doses to keep the inevitable depression at bay.[27]

Withdrawal from pharmaceutical or OTC diet pills is not life-threatening. However, the withdrawing abuser is strongly advised to elicit some medical advice, particularly since more than amphetamine abuse is often involved. Half of all regular users of amphetamines, for instance, are also heavy drinkers.[28] During early withdrawal, depression, lethargy, long periods of sleep, disorientation, and suicidal tendencies are common, and some symptoms may persist for a year.[29] A woman going through withdrawal needs constant assurance that her depression and sense of doom are a normal, and passing, part of getting clean. She also needs someone to share her rediscovery of the fullness of life without drugs.

The story that follows chronicles one woman's twenty-year dependence on diet pills, and their sometimes harrowing effect on her life. Diana's story is important for another reason. Like half the women we interviewed, she is an adult child of an alcoholic parent, an ACA.

There are thirty million adult and young children of alcoholics in this country.[30] They come from all social, ethnic, and religious backgrounds, but there is a stunning commonality to their experi-ence: they grow up amidst emotional chaos and violence. Their lives are a series of family disruptions, with parents arguing, blacked out, hungover or simply not there. Early in life they learn the bitter lesson that no one cares about their needs. They have been called the Forgotten Children.[31]

Although many women from alcoholic homes appear to grow up unscathed, all have been touched by their environment.[32] They are heirs to a constellation of problems. Compared to children of nonalcoholics they have higher incidences of hyperactivity and school problems, higher arrest rates, lower self-esteem, more trouble with intimacy, and more difficulty expressing their needs. In adulthood, they have higher rates of divorce and depression, and a risk of becoming alcoholic that is four times greater than children of nonalcoholic parents.[33,34]

Parental abuse of alcohol takes its toll in every area of a woman's development. In the final chapter we discuss some of the devastating and longlasting effects of sexual abuse on girls. Half of all incest victims are from alcoholic homes and most child molestation is committed under the influence of alcohol.[35]

Most children of alcoholics have witnessed family violence or were themselves abused.[36] Millions of girls grow up believing that violence is an acceptable way of solving family problems, and that violence against women is normal. As adults, these women all too often marry alcoholics and relive the victimization of their childhoods: virtually all battering husbands use alcohol.[37,38]

ACA women learn to ignore their own pain. They have never truly experienced the losses and traumas of their childhood. As children of five, they behaved like thirty. As women of thirty, they feel they are five. They bear the weight of years of delayed and unfelt grief.[39]

In finding ways around this delayed grief, often the delayed grief of generations, ACAs set unrealistically high expectations for themselves; and when they fail, they fall prey to depression and self-recrimination, which often can only be relieved by alcohol or other mood-altering chemicals.[40] As children they typically feel that somehow they are the cause of their parent's drinking. They take upon themselves the burden of keeping everything all right in the family, becoming children without a childhood.[41] As women, they form relationships in which they cater to someone else's needs without admitting needs of their own, thus achieving enmeshment while avoiding intimacy. As mothers, they are often overwhelmed by having to nurture their children, trying to give the nurturing they never got.[42]

The ACA dilemma was completely unrecognized until the late seventies. Until then, children with ACA problems were diagnosed as having everything from manic depression to "adjustment reactions."[43] Now, these children are receiving increased understanding and attention. Articles, books, and TV discussion shows appear regularly. At least one general-audience magazine deals exclusively with ACA issues.[44] Most cities have Twelve Step meetings for teens (Alateen) and for adult children (Alanon, ACA). And while comparatively few studies deal with the special problems of female ACAs, as more and more women come forward with their stories, as Diana has done, that is bound to change.

*   *   *

Diana's Story

We spoke with Diana in the kitchen of her suburban home while upstairs in the family room, her two teenagers and their four friends played pool. When we first met Diana we were struck by her looks. Her dark skin and hair contrast sharply with her light hazel eyes. And we were immediately aware of her warm, upbeat manner. She speaks with the lively pace and expressive animation of a New Yorker. At the time of our interview she had been off pills for seven years.

I was born in New York City in 1938 and I'm an only child. My childhood was filled with impending doom. My father was an alcoholic with an explosive temper. One minute I'd be playing quietly in my room and the next minute there was this bang, yell, boom and my mother would be crying, my father would slam the door, and he'd be gone all evening to the bar across the street. Then I'd lie in bed waiting for him to come home cursing and knocking things over.

My mother was a classic co-alcoholic. My father couldn't hold a job, but Mother never blamed his drinking. It was his "temper" that always got him fired. For most of my childhood he was out of work, so my mother supported us completely. She had a big career as a fashion magazine editor.

She was a nervous, martyred, Jewish mother, one of the early Super Moms—working all day, cooking and housecleaning at night. And sighing and crying about my father this, my father that. "He's such a baby, he's such an animal . . . ." And my father was always angry. It was a grim household. Even the cat slinked around with this frightened look.

It seemed like our lives were always on the verge of falling apart. We never seemed to have any *small* problems. Everything was treated like a catastrophe. So as a child I had no way to put anything into perspective and I couldn't trust my perceptions.

When things came undone, only my successes could hold them together. If I won a swimming race, or played in a girls' concert, everybody was happy for a little while. I became the family heroine—a desperate little girl with a great mission. But if my marks weren't top, if I lost my key or misplaced my comb, if there were dishes in the sink or lint on the floor then Mama could cry and Papa would grow grim and the steel trap of the family would once more choke us all in sadness and despair. That's the child of an alcoholic.

"I spent a lot of time and energy keeping my weight down."

My mother was very ambitious for me. We were lower middle class, but I always went to private schools. When I was twelve I got a scholarship to an exclusive secondary and high school. As soon as I sat down in my first class, I knew that everything about me was wrong—my clothes, my briefcase, the way I moved, the place I lived, everything. The other kids had successful fathers, and mothers who did charity luncheons. I was ashamed of my topsy-turvy background and, in order to flip it, I lied and made up stories. The real difference between them and me was that their homes were quiet and made emotional sense. But I pinned my feeling of being different on material things.

One day when I was thirteen I was sitting in the school cafeteria and I overheard two girls talking. "You know," one of them said, "Diana would be pretty if she lost some weight." That remark burned into me. I figured, maybe if I lose weight they'll all accept me. I went on a diet and lost twenty pounds. I started being popular with boys and that made the girls accept me. So weight became my ticket to acceptance.

"I knew I had found a key to living."

I had never been invited to any school parties but, when I was fifteen, a good-looking boy named Larry invited me to a big fancy Park Avenue bash which many of my classmates were going to. He was part of the school's "in" crowd and this was my big chance. I was going to waltz in on his arm and everyone would just have to accept me. I was so nervous I was shaking. The hostess came toward us with such confidence and poise. I started to say hello but all I could do was stammer. I went to the bar and asked for whiskey. After a few sips I felt better. After two drinks I was comfortable with everyone there. All the fear disappeared.

I knew I had found some key to living. A couple of drinks and I was social and delightful. I was charming. I had confidence and poise. I was good enough. I didn't have to flip my life to make me acceptable. Drinking did the flipping for me. It was the great equalizer.

Larry and I went together for a few years, and then we got engaged. I enrolled in a prestigious East Coast college. I was winning all the prizes and conning other people into believing that I belonged in this rich, successful world. But *I* never believed it. And to take away the sting of feeling always illegitimate I was getting drunk every weekend. I remember once ending up in a hotel with a man I didn't even know, in and out of a blackout.

On my wedding day I got riotously drunk, went into a black-out, threw up, and was sick all night. And for the next three years, things got worse and worse and I drank more and more. I started having affairs and Larry divorced me. The marriage had lasted three years.

"I flaunted my skinniness."

For a while, I drifted from one half-a— secretarial job to another. I went out with stockbrokers and lawyers to fancy East Side night-clubs, but the whole lifestyle seemed hollow and phony and I didn't want it anymore. Then one night a college friend called me and said her homosexual cousin had invited her to go to a bar where men danced together and would I like to go. "I'd love to," I said.

We went into this dingy bar with mafia types guarding the door. You could barely see anything except silhouettes of men holding each other on the dance floor. It was illegal and there were big black curtains on the window. These people were living on the very margins of society and I felt I had come home. It was a tremendous relief, for the first time in my life, not to have to compete in the mainstream of society. And these men didn't treat me like a sex object. I felt appreciated.

I started to lead a very social life in the gay world and my weight got way out of hand. I was up to 130 pounds, twenty pounds more than I wanted to be. One of my new friends, an interior decorator, said, "I've got something that will help you." He took me into his gold and marble bathroom and picked up a big glass jar full of colored pills.

"Put out both your hands," he said. I cupped my two palms together and he filled them with diet pills. I started taking them right there, one a day. They were time-released diet pills—Escatrol. I didn't like them. They made me nervous. They made my mouth dehydrate. They made me feel funny. But they *did* suppress my appetite. And I started to lose weight without even trying. I got down to 110. I flaunted my skinniness.

And the pills did a lot more. I never had to be tired again. I'd set my alarm at seven o'clock, pop a pill, and go back to sleep till 7:30. Then I'd be *awake*. People said, "How do you stay so thin?" I said, "No problem." "How do you party so much?" "No problem." As long as I had my pills, I never had to get tired, depressed, or bored again, even if all I did was pick lint off the carpet. I never had to have another hangover. My pills gave me incredible courage. I had everything licked.

People warned me about having to take bigger and bigger doses, so I'd take the pills during the week and on the weekend I'd cold-turkey it, going through the worst depression and horrible feelings. Come Monday, I'd pop a pill and get a virgin high. I could go way back up. I never had to up my daily dose, not for twenty-two years. I only changed the brand, from Escatrol, to Dexamil, to Dexedrine and finally Didrex.

"I was into pure living . . . and I kept taking speed."

I ran through a large collection of friends' diet pills so I had to develop doctor sources of my own. It was easy in those days before there were triplicate prescription forms. One friend stole a couple of sheets off doctors' prescription pads and wrote his own scrips.

Another turned me on to her speed doctor. All I had to do was tell him I needed something for my weight.

At one of the gay bars I made friends with a young playwright. He let me audition for his first play which was being done off-off-Broadway. Even though I had never acted before, I got the part. All I needed was to pop a diet pill and say my lines. But when I took a pill during the actual performance, I became paralyzed. So when I was in a play, I took diet pills through all the rehearsals, then on opening night I went out on stage crashing.

In the meantime, the sixties were progressing and so was my alcoholism. At twenty-eight I got cirrhosis of the liver and knew I better stay away from alcohol. I discovered LSD and pot. I became a true flower child—fringes, hippie beads, yoga, peace, and love. I lay down in front of the Draft Induction Center and was almost trampled by mounted police. I was a vegetarian, into pure living and against society. But I kept taking my speed, and I soon went back to drinking.

By this time I was on Didrex, my all-time favorite. It wasn't time released so I used to get a nice rush from it. I took a half at a time, every two and a half hours, till three in the afternoon, when I switched to liquor or Quaaludes.

Taking diet pills wasn't a flower child thing to do, so I became secretive about it. We were all being told speed kills, and I was afraid it was going to get tougher and tougher to get it. Then I met a gay doctor who became my friend and my final great source. He prescribed them as needed, every month for years on end. Because he was my sole source, I tried to be a good patient. I had tremendous anxiety—what if he moved, what if he died? Every month I called him, my voice as honeyed as possible. "Oh, Erwin, how *are* you? How's everything in your life? I was just wondering, by the way, if I could have another scrip? Oh, thank you. That would be great. Thank you so much. Thank you." There was a world of drama around that prescription.

When I was twenty-eight I spent a summer in a little community outside San Francisco and I stopped taking diet pills. After five days of crashing I had a release of energy that was so amazing. I remember doing a lot of the things that I used to do on speed, like incessant cleaning, but I did it with a kind of a joy instead of that drivenness I had on speed. I had energy that I couldn't believe and a sense of well-being. Also, I had a tremendous appetite.

"I sat there, flying on speed, saying, 'Relax.'"

I took one look at myself when I got back to New York—I don't think they had any full-length mirrors in Northern California—and saw that I had gained twenty pounds. I was going through a bad period in my life when my career wasn't going anywhere and I didn't know what the next move was. I thought, "Oh sh—, I should go back on diet pills."

I was convinced that I had an insufficient level of adrenalin and that I needed diet pills to function normally. I took them not to get high but to get by. I had been taking them for eight years.

I began studying yoga and got into teaching yoga classes and meditation. I sat there, flying on speed, saying, "Close your eyes, relax, be aware of your breathing, go deep within, feel the inner peace." Everyone said I was the best teacher in the yoga institute, which underlined the sense I had of myself as a fraud.

I was living this fraudulent life, and if you liked or accepted me that was proof I had conned you. I had a strange dissociation from myself because I was preaching one thing and doing another, talking inner peace but feeling none of it. Diet pills enabled me to simulate a life, simulate emotions, simulate activities in which somehow I was not a participant.

"There was an unbelievable relief being back on diet pills."

When I was thirty I got married again and the following month I got pregnant. I went off diet pills and everything else, including meat, sugar, and coffee. I was baking my own bread, and eating huge amounts of natural protein like whole wheat pancakes and homemade peanut butter. I spent the whole day cooking for myself. I never got on a scale. I never went to a doctor either.

I ran into my speed doctor in the Village one day and he said, "Which doctor has let you do this?" I said, "What doctor? I'm not going to a doctor." He said, "You must have gained fifty pounds!" I said, "I don't know, I'm not weighing myself." He said, "It's dangerous to the baby if you have fat in the birth canal." I hadn't heard that one before. He took me up to his office and I weighed in at 165 pounds. I had gone from 113 to 165, from a size five to a size fourteen.

My husband and I tried to have the baby at home but after fifty hours of labor, we called my speed doctor and he got me into the hospital. I had natural childbirth in the hospital and my baby was born and I nursed her. I went on a diet right away trying to get my weight down. I went from 156 down to 130, but I couldn't bring it down any further. I always had trouble around 130. I simply couldn't get below that.

Nursing my daughter was the most important and the best part of our relationship. Looking down at her head at my breast, feeling the tug of her sucking, it was pure joy. I would lie there grooving on the whole experience, its sensation, its meaning. I think it was the only time in my life I had ever relaxed.

But when she was six months old, I felt I couldn't go on any longer without *something*. Taking care of a baby was terribly hard for me. It took everything I had just to get through each day. I had no friends where we lived and felt totally alone, lost, and depressed. I had been off diet pills for fifteen months, the longest period of abstinence since I had started taking them. I started taking Didrex again and nursing at the same time.

I looked at my little daughter closely, all the time watching to see, was she different? Anytime she cried, any strange movement or tone, I thought, "Oh my God, is it the Didrex?" I kept checking and rechecking it, thinking, "She is more cranky; then again, no, I'm imagining it." Back and forth like that all day.

There was an unbelievable relief in being back on diet pills. I thought, "Thank God I don't have to take care of my own life anymore. It's just too damn hard."

My life was really disintegrating at that time. My husband and I had huge, violent fights. At these times, I'd go into the hall into this little cubicle with an incinerator and people's garbage. I'd just sit there on the floor, with people's garbage bags around me, and cry. We split up for several months, then got back together. He always blamed my diet pills. Once he took my pills and poured them down the drain.

I made an emergency call to my doctor but he said he was booked for the day and couldn't see me. So I went to his office anyway with my two-year-old daughter and sat on the steps outside for three hours waiting for a scrip. I had big stones in my pockets so when he weighed me I'd be overweight and he would give me the same strong pills. At last he saw me and I got my Didrex. I still remember that relief.

Around that time I discovered I was three months pregnant. I had been on speed the whole time. I think I was numb to the implications of that. Actually, I was, thanks to the pills, numb to pretty much everything. My husband was horrified. I think at this point any love he had left for me froze up. He said, "You have got to get off them."

"I felt that I was talking and moving too fast."

We had moved back to Manhattan to a residential hotel and I rented a separate room where I could crash. The crash and the withdrawal were much worse than before. I slept for a whole month and was unable to do anything, just crash out, day after day after day, finally getting back to some semblance of normality. My relationship with my husband was very bad. We barely spoke at all. There was a continual hard silence between us.

I got through that pregnancy, drinking a little, smoking some marijuana, but off the pills. My son's birth was easier than my daughter's had been. I could feel great waves of love for him, but they were overshadowed by fear—fear about my competence as a mother. I had a newborn infant and a two-year-old baby in diapers and on a bottle. From the moment I got up until the moment I got to sleep and several times during the night there were these babies crying, needing me, needing me. My husband took tremendous responsibility with these infants. But nothing was enough. I had the feeling during the day that I was going crazy. I counted the hours from the moment I got up—how many hours till this day ends? I didn't think I would live through it. And in the back of my mind, "If only I could take Didrex. At least it will be a little better." Every night I whimpered with relief, "I got through the day." Then I had to get through the night, because babies get up. There was no relief.

After nursing my son for three weeks we went to visit a friend at his country house and I thought, "I can't go on any more. I can't get through this day." I had taken the pills with me, even though I was off them. Even if I was off them for six months I kept a stash with me, and a stash at home in case anything should happen to my purse. At the country house I thought, "Should I take a pill? You mustn't. You're nursing. He's a three-week-old baby. You can't do that!" I took a half.

The next day I took a pill and it was a little better, but not a hell of a lot better. After we got back home I stayed off speed, counting the days till I stopped nursing. I had nursed my first child for two years. This time, I decided I would hold out for three months. I thought, "He doesn't really need to be nursed that long. I can't do it this time. Just can't." I made it through three months, counting the days. Then I put him on a bottle, on formula, and went back to pills.

Again I experienced that unbelievable relief, being able to sink into the strong arms of this drug and have it carry me through the day. Around this time my husband and I both discovered cocaine. He did a lot more than I did. He liked to get amped up at night, when I'd be crashing. We were going every which way. We had a big blowout and he threw my pills down the drain again. I got another scrip again.

I brought my two young children out to Southern California for a summer. I felt that I was talking and moving too fast. I went off pills for six months, then my weight went up, and I knew I needed them even in mellow California.

I went to a doctor friend of my parents who said, "Oh, I don't believe in those pills." That put me into a real panic. I called my doctor in New York and he said, "You're very, very lucky because I'm licensed in both states." He was able to write me a scrip for Didrex on a California pad and mail it to me and I filled it.

Then, one day I called him and he said, "I can't. They're cracking down in New York and counting every pill written on triplicate. Anyway, they're not good for you." He said that after twenty years.

"It's not something I want to stay on."

I went doctor shopping. I got into that junkie nightmare of being without a source, taking other kinds of speed, trying to find the right dose, always trying to connect. Finally I went back to the friend of the family doctor and did one of those drug-addict snow jobs: "I've just given up smoking," I said. Actually, I had just gone *back* to smoking—so the first thing out of my mouth was a lie. "I'm gaining a lot of weight because of quitting smoking. I've *got* to have them. I'm very depressed, too. Just help me over these first two months. It's very temporary. It's not something I want to stay on." I knew the sheer energy of my need would overcome his objections. I won him over. He even threw in a Valium prescription. I said, "Why are you giving me these?" He said, "To help you calm down."

I looked at the speed scrip and gasped, "That's half the dose I asked you for." He said, "Oh, you don't need that much." I made him rewrite the prescription.

I was actually singing and dancing on the way home, as if the greatest victory in my whole life was this prescription in my hand. That was in October.

On January 20th the American hostages were coming home from Iran. I had been watching them all day on television. By evening they were out of Iran free and I was so drunk from a couple of glasses of brandy I couldn't focus on the TV set. I had totally lost my capacity to hold liquor. My husband did an imitation of what I was like drunk: reeling around the room, slurring, bumping into things. On two drinks. It scared me so much, I called Alcoholics Anonymous.

Before my first AA meeting I took a diet pill, a couple of lines of cocaine, and a half a Valium to calm down. The woman who drove me to the meeting asked, "Are you on any drugs?" I said, "I don't think that's any of your business. I'm here for alcohol. If you have any problem with that I can just turn around and go home." She said, "Okay, okay."

She introduced me to another woman saying, "This is her first day." This new woman gave me a warm smile and asked, "How do you like sobriety?"

I said, "Sobriety?" and gulped.

"I had been a hostage and now I was free."

At the second meeting they read from a book: "Some of us have tried to hold on to our old ideas and the result was nil until we let go absolutely." I got this neon flash in my mind: *drugs*. For the first time in my life it occurred to me that my need to take the diet pills was an old idea I had never questioned. I always assumed that I really needed them.

At home I made a color-coded chart on graph paper of all the drugs I had taken from age nineteen, different colors for different drugs. I looked at the brilliant colors all over the chart and two things were obvious. One, I was a drug addict; I was chemically dependent. Not a day, except for the nine months pregnant with my first child, had I been off mood-altering chemicals. Two, my drug of choice was obviously this bar of red that went right down the page. It was: "Oh, that's the one!" I hadn't *known* it was my primary drug.

It was always: reach under the bed for my purse in the morning the moment I wake up, take out this little vial, pop the pill into my mouth, then go on with my life. The diet pills were invisible, except when there was a crisis, like going to triplicate, or my doctor saying, "No more prescriptions," or my husband saying, "Down the drain," or finding out I'm pregnant.

On Saturday as I lay in bed crashing for the weekend I knew I had to get off everything. I had gotten off alcohol three days before. Monday came and I didn't take a pill. That day the hostages came home to America and every store sold yellow ribbons. I bought one and stuck it on my rearview mirror. Looking at it, I knew it was for me, too. I had been a hostage and now I was free.

I haven't had a drug since.

"You may gain weight and that's going to be okay."

When I quit, we had no health insurance so I couldn't afford an alcohol and drug rehab program, but at one hospital the program director said I could sit in on certain groups on an informal basis and I did that for several days. I saw films and talked about the disease of chemical dependency. I felt I was fighting for my life, with their help.

At an early meeting of Alcoholics Anonymous I saw a plaque on the wall, "When all else fails, try following directions." I had always done everything my own way, but I couldn't do this. I knew nothing about sobriety.

They told me to get a sponsor. I got a sponsor and told her my life story. She listened quietly for three hours and had just one question for me: "What if you gain weight? Are you going back on pills?"

For the first time I faced that gritty question and made a commitment to myself: "You may gain weight and that's going to be okay. Whatever happens, you don't go back on diet pills."

I carried sixty pills in that plastic vial with the orange triplicate label for six months, clean and sober. Then I put them in the cabinet. Later I put them in a strong box with all kinds of mood-changing chemicals. A little codeine. A little Valium. A regular drug store.

When I was over a year clean and sober I told my sponsor and she said, "Throw those damn pills out." Like me, my husband hadn't taken anything for a year, but he had the same stashing instinct. As I was throwing the contents of a bottle in the toilet he said, "Stop! We can give those to someone!" Our attitude was, "Who will inherit the family jewels?"

I took bottle after bottle and threw all the Didrex out—they made this huge foam in the toilet bowl that was just marvelous to look at—and then flushed it.

I weighed 132 when I got sober. A year later I had gained only six pounds so it was obvious that I didn't need diet pills to control my weight. After two years of sobriety I quit smoking for good and went up to 145. I felt that was going out of control and went to Overeaters Anonymous and got back to 132.

Becoming sober, for me, is like the onion. Underneath alcohol were drugs. Beneath drugs was food. And beneath the food are the issues of who am I and is it okay for me to be here, and what did it mean to have a father who was an alcoholic and out of control? And a mother who was anxious, overachieving and perfectionistic? I've been sorting that out in individual therapy, still working on the onion, that whole addiction structure, peeling, peeling, healing, healing.

"I spent twenty-six years numbing my feelings."

Once in the first year I wanted desperately to take a pill. I called up another recovering speed freak and said, "I don't feel I'm going anywhere." She said, "What's missing? Whatever it is, that's what made you take speed." We got it down to scary feelings I wanted to run from. The hardest thing for me was *not* to do something, just stand there. "And what did the speed do?" she asked. Speed made me feel I was moving when I was only running in place. Whenever I felt anxious I wanted to run. Once I faced that, the fantasy about speed as savior and solution was over. I was learning that the only way out was *through*.

My feelings used to be so extreme, I was always shaking angry, crying sad, dying lonely, or crazy giddy and ecstatic, and I was guilty for feeling that way. All this resurfaced after I got off drugs. Today my feelings are not so black and white. They're even a barometer for me.

I spent twenty-six years numbing my feelings. Imagine someone who spent twenty-six years in bed trying to work out. Imagine how sore the muscles would get, how they'd spasm and hurt, how long it would take to give them strength and tone. But after a while, it's wonderful to move and lift them and coordinate them and feel their vitality.

Sobriety has been progressive. More and more, I can listen to myself and trust what I hear. Even when I feel distress there's an underlying well-being that I never had in my life.

People say AA stands for Altered Attitudes. I've found I can alter my attitude by sharing my feelings. The sharing is the work out. The sharing is the healing.

"I feel good inside my own skin."

I never understood love. I thought it was doing, jumping through hoops. I thought being a mother meant being on call all the time. I couldn't stand that and I felt like a failure. Then I sponsored my first AA newcomer. I sat with her, listening to her life story—tears in her eyes, embarrassed and scared. "What am I going to do for her," I groaned to myself. In one moment I realized, all I had to do was be there for her and that was easy and it felt good. Then I could start to let myself be there for my own children.

It's taken years to get over the guilt with my children but this year I was able to sit down with them for breakfast, morning after morning, and *be there*. I began to enjoy them. Then I saw how I had missed what motherhood could give *me*. *I* had never been nourished by it before. It was always energy out. Now the energy comes in, particularly from my family. Things are often painful and full of conflict, but they're energizing, nourishing, healing. I never imagined motherhood could be those things. I always thought it was just work.

With this, I've gotten close to other women. When I first got clean and sober I liked to brag, "I have no problem with other women," but the fact is that I had few real friendships with women and no sense of the *enjoyment* of women friends. I think I couldn't stand the mirror image of other women. At first, I thought I didn't like them. Underneath that, I found that I was afraid they wouldn't like me. Underneath *that*, I didn't like myself.

Today, the closeness I feel with other women is one of the most intense, exciting, and rewarding things in my life. I've gone through the pain and fear to the joy of women friends. Tonight I'm going out with about six women to a Chinese restaurant and then maybe a meeting. We're recovering people, nonrecovering, straight, gay, married, single, in our twenties, thirties, and forties. It's something I haven't done since high school—be with a bunch of women. It's come with my accepting and liking myself.

After five years of being sober I realized that my marriage had stayed drunk. My husband and I went to marriage counseling and started changing years of the old alcoholic dynamics: controlling, rescuing, playing victim, and—above all—not talking. Today we can share. I can say what I need or feel and so can he without playing all the games around feelings and needs. After a year of counseling, we get very silly and affectionate together and we have a sense of adventure. So even our marriage is getting sober.

The things I thought I needed speed for I have on my own—a strong spiritual life, interesting work, lots of energy. I feel good inside my own skin. The great gift is coming to myself. Even that poor desperate crazy creature I used to be. I was inside her. I know now how she felt. I've gone back and felt the feelings I never had then. To others she may have been a desperate spectacle. To me she was a lost, confused, sick person in need of help. I really love her.

6

Painkillers
Tricia's Story

Killing the Pain of Life

When pain strikes, we reach for a pill. Even minor pain is something we don't have time for. We are trained from the crib that if we hurt, there's a pill that will make us feel better. We chug down more than *nineteen billion* aspirin a year.[1] We have become so used to taking something for pain—and so sure that what we take actually works—experiments show that thirty-five percent of us actually get relief even if we are given placebos.[2]

Our pursuit of pain-free living has made the highly addictive narcotic analgesics some of the most widely used of all controlled drugs. In 1980, one narcotic painkiller—codeine—was an ingredient in nearly fifteen percent of all controlled prescriptions. Of the twenty most frequently prescribed controlled drugs, eight contained a narcotic painkiller.[3]

Women are especially prone to being given a prescription painkiller. They are far more likely than men to visit family doctors or internists, and they are often brought into contact with medical practitioners because of premenstrual syndrome, menstruation problems, and giving birth. One doctor estimates that ninety-five percent of births are medicated to some degree, with Demerol being one of the most widely used narcotic painkillers.[4] Demerol, however, can depress the mother's breathing and interfere with the unborn child's supply of oxygen.[5]

The narcotic painkillers are either extracted from opium or are synthesized compounds that act like opium in the body. These opiates include morphine, codeine, and the brand-name drugs Dilaudid, Demerol, Methadone, Darvon, Talwin and Percodan.

They are all extraordinarily effective at blocking pain, and the legitimacy of their use with cancer patients and the severely injured is beyond dispute. But five percent of Americans—nearly nine million people—use these drugs for nonmedical purposes.[6]

The opiates are abused on such a scale because they do more than take away pain. They also take away fear, ease worry, relieve anxiety and soothe the feelings of inferiority that plague so many women. Day-to-day concerns vanish, or simply become meaningless. The lonely are comforted, the bored distracted, and everything comes up roses.

Though opiates may tranquilize a woman's mind, they neverthe-less vex her body. They decrease her sex hormone levels, and sex drive, and in some cases cause an alteration of her menstruation cycle. Opiates depress her central nervous system and her breathing, and contract the pupils of her eyes. With even moderate doses she becomes constipated, sometimes dangerously so. In high doses the opiates produce coma or convulsion. Children born to mothers who continued to use these painkillers while pregnant may have become addicts in the womb and, in their first week of life, they will be viewing their world through the convulsive agonies of narcotic withdrawal.[7]

Nearly all the opiates have a history of being considered safe when they were first introduced. As with heroin itself, each seemed to be the wonder drug that, unlike the wonder drugs that went before it, finally promised relief from pain without the dread of addiction.

• Morphine, extracted from opium in 1814, was thought for years to be relatively harmless. In the early 1900s society women were reported using it to "calm their shattered nerves," and "allay their ennui."[8] At the turn of the century, physicians prescribed it to "cure" alcoholism, a practice that continued among some doctors well into the middle of this century.[9] When heroin was invented, some physicians used it to "cure" morphine addiction. At present, morphine-caused deaths are listed as heroin/morphine overdoses. Twenty percent of known female drug deaths are heroin/morphine overdoses.

- Codeine, the most widely used natural opiate, is considered a fairly weak drug with only a moderate potential for physical dependence. It is currently used in over forty cold, cough, and pain medicines.[10] As a contributing cause in emergency room visits, codeine affects more women than men.[11] It ranks as one of the five most frequently listed substances in reports of drug deaths among women.[12]

- Methadone, first synthesized in 1943 and named Dolophine in honor of Adolf Hitler, is currently given to cancer patients to reduce pain and to heroin addicts as a substitute for heroin in federally-controlled treatment programs. Seventy percent of female Methadone users suffer from abnormal menses.[13] In some major cities, deaths from Methadone overdose have outnumbered deaths from heroin overdose.[14] Methadone is a factor in four percent of female drug deaths.[15]

- Darvon, closely related to Methadone, has become the object of widespread abuse in recent years. It is the second most commonly prescribed controlled substance, and is second only to the barbiturates as a prescription drug linked to drug deaths.[16] In 1984, a survey of hospitals in twenty-seven metropolitan areas listed Darvon as a contributing cause in nearly two thousand emergency room incidents, with women outnumbering men two to one. Women also outnumber men two to one in Darvon-related deaths.[17]

All the opiates are capable of producing profound tolerance, which means it takes ever-increasing doses to get the same effect. Since tolerance to one opiate will produce tolerance to all, a woman switching from Demerol to Darvon to Percodan to "control" her use is playing a losing game.[18]

Inevitably, chronic use of any opiates in any combination leads to psychological and physical addiction. Once that point is reached, the user must continue taking her drug, not so much for the pleasure it once produced, but because stopping means withdrawing.

While withdrawal from the painkillers is rarely life-threatening, it can be painful and disabling. As with most drugs, women attempting to get clean are advised to do so with medical supervision, particularly since many women dependent on painkillers are also dependent on—and will be withdrawing from—alcohol or sedatives.[19]

Opiate withdrawal symptoms usually begin at the time of the next scheduled dose, and include restlessness, anxiety, chills, nausea, muscle twitching, abdominal cramps, and depression. With some of the opiates, gooseflesh gives the skin the look of plucked turkey, hence the phrase *cold turkey*. Withdrawal symptoms usually disappear within five to ten days.

Withdrawal from Darvon deserves special attention. In many ways it resembles the more serious withdrawal from the sedatives and may include hallucinations, confusion, delusions and seizures.[20]

Withdrawal from the opiates is ideally attempted in a residential treatment center. Such centers do more than oversee withdrawal symptoms. Their carefully planned programs often include lectures, group therapy and individual assignments, which can help inform the recovering substance abuser about the underlying reasons for her chemical dependency.

As Tricia's story demonstrates, a well-run treatment program offers a nonthreatening environment in which a woman can explore and develop relationship skills. Interacting with other people who are committed to the same goals can help a woman look at her drug abuse with compassion and understanding, especially in the early weeks of sobriety, when guilt is often keenly felt. And, finally, a supportive and nurturing group can be essential in enhancing that most critical foundation of a woman's sobriety: her sense of self-worth.

Tricia's participation in a rehabilitation group for addicted professionals sheds light on an aspect of painkiller abuse rarely spoken about—addiction among nurses. Nearly four percent of nurses are dependent on narcotics, a rate that is up to fifty percent higher than in the general population.[21] Some reasons for this high rate are poignantly illustrated by Tricia's story—nurses' easy access to the drugs; the physical stresses of nursing, including staggered shifts and long days; and the emotional ordeal of working with the sick and dying. But equally important is the attitude of Tricia and other nurses toward legal painkillers—unlike street drugs, these "medicines" are an acceptable source of relief.[22]

We had a long, if sporadic, relationship with painkiller "medicine." For years, no trip to the dentist was complete without a codeine prescription. And any visit to a doctor that involved pain was always good for a scrip of Darvon. We really thought we needed them, if only for a day or two. In a nine-year period we must have bought several hundred pills. We probably used no more than a few dozen, but it was comforting to know they were right there in our medicine chest. Like all druggies, stashing was part of our habit. Now, in sobriety, when a dentist or doctor kindly offers us a narcotic painkiller, we decline. We say we'll call them if we need something.

In the past six years, we haven't called once.

* * *

Tricia's Story

We first met Tricia when she was four months pregnant, and she looked happy and radiant. She wore a patterned, loose fitting dress and her brown hair was tied back in a ponytail. When she laughed, which was fairly often, she held back nothing. Her eyes sparkled and her whole body gently shook. When we began our session, her son, an adorable three-year-old, kept interrupting with various jobs for his mother. Tricia was a model of patience. Finally, he parked himself in front of the TV and Tricia told her story.

I was born in Washington state in 1952, the oldest girl of six children. My dad was a dental technician and he was always getting better jobs, which meant moving around a lot. We moved from city to city and state to state. I went to three kindergartens, two first grades, and three second grades.

It was real difficult to grow up like that. I learned early on how to make quick superficial relationships. And how to keep everything looking okay on the outside even though I was falling apart on the inside.

My father was an alcoholic, the kind who never drank at home and was sober as a judge all week. But every Friday night he'd go out and get rip-roaring drunk. When he got home at three in the morning, everybody knew about it. He'd park the car at the top of a tree or something.

My mother was a great enabler, one of these very passive "well-what-do-you-think-we-should-do-honey?" type women. When Dad got drunk and acted like a crazy person I stood between the two of them. At a young age I could take care of things.

I think from the time I was born I had this drive: everything had to be perfect. And in an alcoholic home nothing is perfect. I made sure the house was clean, I made dinners every night. I took care of my brothers and sisters. And like a lot of adult children of alcoholics, I never learned how to play or relax. I was real thin because I was on the edge all the time.

I wouldn't bring friends home from school because the morning dishes would still be on the table and the house would look like it had been ransacked. So I'd march into the house and just start cleaning.

I didn't take drugs in a serious way till I was an adult, even though I grew up in the sixties—when if someone didn't pass out from something it wasn't Monday. I tried to smoke marijuana and I fell asleep. My high school boyfriend was great for drugs. He figured out you could make money on this and he went off and running. To me drugs were something good kids didn't do.

"I thought, this is a good way to go."

After I finished high school, in L.A., my family moved back to Washington. I stayed in L.A. and went to nursing school. On Friday night I'd get rip-roaring drunk, but you'd never know it. One night a girlfriend and I are pulled over by some cops. They give her a drunk test and take her in. They shined the light in my face and said, "We'd like you to follow us to the station so you can take your girlfriend home." Well, I'm as drunk as she is but I looked okay.

After I graduated from nursing school I moved to a smaller city. I met Joel and we started living together. He bugged me to marry him, but I wasn't sure. In a few months I started working in an emergency room. Within a year I was in charge, which was just typical. And that's where I met up with painkillers.

I was the kind of person who didn't take medicine, not even an aspirin for a headache. But while I was in college I broke my foot. My doctor said, "I'm going to give you a prescription for pain medicine." I didn't want it, but when I got home I realized this throbbing was not going to go away and I called him and said, "All I can think about is the pain in my foot." He said, "Well, take the prescription." I took Tylenol No. 3 with codeine every day for two weeks. I thought, this is a good way to go. So here it is, two years later, I'm working in an ER, and I realize it's really easy to take things out of hospitals if you have half a brain.

"I bet I won't be lonely if I take this pill."

The first time, I remember, was when I got some Percodan for a patient and then found out he was allergic to them. Well, I'd already taken them out of the little unit-dose packages and if I had thrown them away—wasted them, as we called it—I'd have to have another RN sign for them and witness me flushing them down the toilet. So I thought, I'll take these two pills home. No big deal. You never know when a friend might need a pain medication.

But I *had* no friends at this point in life. I was really lonely. Joel worked at night and I had no one to talk to. I remember thinking the day that I took the Percodan home, "I bet I wouldn't be so lonely if I take this pill. I'll bet this will make me not care so much about the loneliness and the isolation." And I took it and I was right! I didn't care if I ever saw another human being.

So it started real innocent. A pill here, a pill there. It was always one of the painkillers, like codeine or Percodan. I found I could tolerate a lot of drugs and not look like I was on anything.

For the first year I made sure that all the drugs I took from the ER were legitimate waste. I didn't steal medicine that was meant for patients. I had really high values. But I was obsessed about drugs right from the start. I would go to work hoping, "Maybe tonight we'll need to waste some pain medication."

A year after I started using, Joel and I got married. I stayed off pills for a couple of months. I didn't even think about them. Joel didn't take drugs either, but he drank like a fish. I married an alcoholic. We were a great team.

A year after we were married I discovered my father had liver cancer. It's not a real painful form of cancer, but he was being given Dilaudid pills a hundred at a shot. The man had no pain at all, but doctors feel better if they give you something to get you high. So I started taking them.

"I realized this was not normal."

At first, they were just out in the open. But my brother, who's a heroin addict, found them so my dad started hiding them. I found them. I gave up drinking because I realized you don't have to have a hangover if you take pain pills. I never had another hangover. Never had to worry about it again. Little did I know you have to go through withdrawals if you stay on them long enough. Oh God. That was the worst. But, I took my dad's pain pills, and there was an unlimited supply. My use became very heavy. It was a daily thing.

The minute I got up I took two. By noon they're wearing off, take two again. And in the evening take two more. Then if I was lucky I could fall asleep by ten or eleven. I got wired on pain medication. I'd be up for days.

By this time, with all the Dilaudid I was taking, I realized this was not normal. There was this very loud voice in my head saying, "Normal people don't do this, they don't take this quantity of medication."

I looked for ways to stop my drug use. I decided if I had a swimming pool my life would be better and I wouldn't care so much that I was isolated. I got the pool put in, and after three months it wasn't fun anymore. So then I told Joel I needed to get pregnant. "Joel, I think the reason I take so many drugs is that I need something more in my life. I need a kid. I want a baby." That was going to stop everything.

So I got pregnant and I stopped using. I knew I had to be really careful those first three months. Then I knew I had a good three or four months in the middle of a pregnancy—God, listen to this—I thought, this is good for the baby to have these drugs in its system. And then I knew the last two months I had to be off drugs or the child could be born addicted. So I stayed clean for like three or four months during my whole pregnancy.

I worked up until the seventh month. And then I figured I wasn't going to be able to still be at work where I had access and not take drugs. But even in those last couple of months there were times when I would get a prescription for cough medicine or something.

When I delivered Joe I just knew I was going to be punished for all this rotten behavior. I deserved to have a defective child. And when he was born healthy and gorgeous and just perfect, I just knew he would become sick and die.

"Pills weren't going to do it anymore."

Every little thing that went wrong with him made me frantic. I would rush him to the pediatrician every day, knowing he was going to die. And it would all be my fault. Just imagine this feeling. I had this child who was the sun and the moon and he's going to be taken away from me. For two weeks I breastfed him and was very careful about what I took. I slept with my hand on his chest to make sure he wouldn't stop breathing. Then Joel started doing cocaine.

Joel found out he could do cocaine and drink and it was wonderful. So I started doing cocaine. I didn't like cocaine. I thought it was just real obnoxious. But it was better than downers. And definitely better than booze. So why not do cocaine? I had to do something, for God's sake.

The poor baby was miserable. I was neurotic all the time. The pediatrician kept saying, "Tricia, will you calm down. He may be colicky and have diarrhea, but he's gaining on weight and he's fine."

The baby really kept me occupied for two months. When he was ten weeks old I went back to work. In the four months I had been away from the hospital my disease had progressed to where I started right in shooting morphine. Pills weren't going to do it anymore. In four weeks I was taking twenty to thirty milligrams of morphine a day, three times the amount a patient would get. I'd spend hours in the hospital bathrooms. I didn't even bother trying to take care of sick people.

Weekends were a bitch. I tried to take enough supplies home, but I couldn't control how fast I shot up. No matter how hard I tried, whatever I took home would be gone by Sunday morning. I'd start withdrawing twelve to fourteen hours after my last dose, so Sundays were just hell.

I'd be real nervous and anxious. I'd shake as if I were freezing and I'd be sweating at the same time. The cramps in my legs and arms would hit and I'd have awful diarrhea. I'd go to bed Sunday morning, but I couldn't sleep.

"I just knew I was the only nurse addict in the world."

The only thing that would stop the withdrawal was another dose of drugs. Monday morning I'd rush to work an hour early and ask to do the narcotics count. It was horrible. It was such a horrible thing to live through. I had gone back to work in July and by October I was stealing a hundred milligrams of morphine a day. I still wasn't stealing the patients' meds because their piddly amounts weren't going to do a thing for me. What's four milligrams? It takes twenty for me to feel. The top of my hand, where I really abused a vein, was purple.

By this time I'm going into work knowing the minute I walk in they're going to drag me away with handcuffs. The hospital had to know what was going on. I just knew I was the only nurse addict in the world, let alone my hospital. There was no one for me to talk to, nowhere for me to go. There were drug rehab centers, but I knew my license would be taken away if I went.

I knew I had to quit the hospital. I submitted a resignation in October, '81. I knew I had to get off drugs. There was just no option. I had a seven-month-old child who I knew was going to be affected by it. And that was always a real motivating thought for me, that my son would grow up with an impaired parent just like I did.

By the time I submitted my resignation Joel knew I was shooting up. He found syringes around the house and he started confronting me. Well he's drinking like a fish and he doesn't have a whole lot to say about whether I'm taking drugs or not. We had those fights. You know, "If you stop taking drugs, I'll stop drinking." "If you stop drinking, I'll stop taking drugs." We both knew the other was not going to stop. Not on our own, anyway.

When I submitted my resignation the hospital asked me to stay on two more weeks. They were doing an investigation on the missing pain medicine and they had narrowed it down to me.

On my last day at work the Director of Nurses called me in and said, "Tricia, we have some problems with the drug records." I was so fed up with my life I just wanted to confess to everything. I confessed to things I hadn't done. I confessed to killing Jimmy Hoffa!

This poor director is sitting there, listening to me confess to one felony after another. She's trying to shut me up. Finally, she says, "I don't think we want to press criminal charges. I don't think that would do you any good and it certainly isn't going to change anything that happened here. I think what I'm going to do is call Consumer Affairs and we'll try to handle it administratively. It will be up to them but I will recommend they just handle it through the Board of Registered Nurses. There'll be no criminal charge with the cops or the Drug Enforcement Agency.''

I went home and told Joel, "The jig's up. I just got busted." When Consumer Affairs called me weeks down the line, I told the policewoman who took the deposition, "I did it, I'm a rotten worthless human being, take my license because I don't deserve to be a nurse." She said, "You certainly have a lot of remorse, Tricia, and I think you're real motivated to get help. Most nurses that come in front of me don't admit they have a problem and never admit they did what we accuse them of doing. This is your first time in front of me. I really will be surprised if I ever see you again. I don't have any trouble making this a probation thing. I'm not going to revoke your license."

I swore off drugs. That was the end. I called my sister who works in a pharmacy and told her what had happened. She brought me bottles of painkillers, things like Darvon, that have just enough stuff in them to get me over the worst of withdrawing. I called a drug rehab center and started outpatient counseling. Six months later Joel stops drinking and things are going along swimmingly.

I went to some NA [Narcotics Anonymous] meetings occasionally. Then I graduated myself and went on my own. I stayed clean for a year and then I went back to work in an Intermediate Care Facility. I had to tell them when I was hired that I was a recovering addict on probation, but that was all in the past. I was never going to steal pills again!

I went to group meetings for addicted doctors and nurses. I was very serious about counseling. I was very serious about getting clean and being content with myself, but I didn't have a clue as to what the Twelve-Step Program was about. And I certainly wasn't going to come to believe in anything except my own power which kept me surviving all these years. So I went along my merry way and just kept control and, you know, pushed the river.

I was working twelve-hour night shifts and still trying to be up in the morning. My son was almost two and at that stage where I could have just clobbered him. He was real active and I was just trying to stay halfway awake, getting two or three hours of sleep every day.

"I realized I couldn't stop."

About this time, my babysitter's husband got cancer. They were Italian and they barely spoke English and they didn't drive. So I would take her husband to the doctor, get his prescription and give him the pills.

I told my counselor, "This is a real uncomfortable position for me to be in. Here I have an addiction problem and I'm helping this guy who has more pills than Upjohn." She said, "This is a very difficult situation but I think you can continue to work with him. This will be a great opportunity for you to exert control." Control! Get real. Well, even if she hadn't said it, that's probably what I would have heard anyway.

I decided I could stay awake more if I started taking pills again. Just occasionally, only when I'm at work. While I wasn't working I wouldn't use. So when I gave the medicine to my babysitter's husband, I took a few pills off the top. And I'm back to being supernurse, buzzing around, getting everything done in five minutes.

That was a time of truth for me. I realized I couldn't stop. I knew I had no control over this drug, and that scared me to death. If I could be that wrong about me and drug addiction, then I must have been wrong about a lot of things. I went from a real cocky smart a— kid out of nursing school who figured she knew everything to somebody who was totally incapable of making any decisions.

Within six months I'm back to my old dosages. Huge amounts of pills. My babysitter's husband got real sick, went into the hospital and I decide that's it, I've got to stop taking drugs. I go through another withdrawal, the worst ever. My hair fell out, I had killer cramps in every muscle of my body, and diarrhea so bad I couldn't eat anything. I lost twenty pounds in a week. I was sick, and I was scared.

"Within a couple of weeks I'm ripping off pills by the handful."

What made it worse was the depression and self-loathing that comes with the withdrawal. As I lay in bed dying I used to say, "You deserve this Tricia. You are a horrendous person for doing this."

Joel took care of me as I withdrew, and I hated it. That somebody had to be running around trying to get chicken broth in *me*. But the memory of withdrawal, that tremendous feeling of being sick and dependent, was always good for six months of sobriety.

After about seven months of being clean, the neighbor's out of the hospital and he's back on pain medication. Here we go again. This time he's got Methadone. I found out that Methadone is as good as Dilaudid. I started taking Methadone and Percodan, every day for three to four months. I got magnificently strung out again. Then the guy died.

I am still not going to steal from the hospital, so I had to get my pills from outside, from doctors. I went to four or five doctors every week, lying about pains I didn't have, telling them I lost the prescription they just gave me. I was so sick of doing it, I couldn't stand looking at myself again. It wasn't even important what was happening to me physically. Emotionally it was killing me. To have to do this. To have to lower myself like this, just to get drugs.

And being a mother made me feel even guiltier. I felt that a kid had to have a good mother. A father didn't have to be depended on. But a mom had to be what she says she's going to be: perfect. I had this picture of a perfect mother, and I knew I was far from it. I used to say to Joel at night, "It's the only job I've every really, really tried my very best at and have not been able to get above inadequate."

But at my job I was still a whiz. And now supernurse gets offered a position back in the ER, with all the drugs I could ever want right at my fingertips. Within a couple of weeks I'm ripping off pills by the handful. I was a wild woman. I just completely reverted. I was stealing and using such huge quantities of pills that I knew I was going to get busted again. You know, the perfect ending to a perfect life.

"Dear God, now I'm withdrawing after a month."

One weekend a nurse asked me about a discrepancy on the narcotics record. I knew that was it. I lied like crazy. I told her I had no idea about it and left. They called me all weekend from the hospital. I knew my butt was in the ringer again. I was going to be fired. They were going to take me to the Consumer Affairs and I couldn't live through that again, I just couldn't.

I went to my counselor. For six months we had been talking about what it was like growing up in an alcoholic household. That day she looked at me and said, "You know, we can talk about your childhood till the cows come home. Your problem is, you have a primary disease. It's called drug addiction. And if you don't start working on it, it's going to kill you." She told me that the best thing for me—nurse, caretaker, controller—would be to go into an inpatient treatment program and learn how to be taken care of.

I said, "Yeah, one day I'll do that." But I couldn't ever imagine my doing that. Taking a month off for me was not in the cards. I would give my husband a month off. Or my son by all means. But not me. A lot of women think that way: "I'll drive you anywhere you want to go, but I'm too ill to drive me around the block." Or, "Who's going to take care of the kids? Is my husband going to leave me?" We're convinced we're the only person who can take care of all these things.

So there I am, July, 1986, knowing I'm about to be busted and having to go through withdrawal again. I used to go three months before I got hooked. Dear God, now I'm withdrawing after a month.

That was where I definitely reached bottom. I didn't need to be seventy years old, or wind up in jail, or lose everything. I had lost myself. No matter what I had, the house and the pool and everything didn't matter anymore. Even my kid didn't mean anything.

So I called my counselor and cried, "I give up, I finally give up. I can't live like this anymore. Get me into a treatment program." And she said, "Good, that sounds like surrender to me." She called the Grainger Treatment Center the next morning. There wasn't even time for me to say, "Well maybe I could make it on my own one more time."

"I started learning from everyone and everything."

When they admitted me, they asked what I wanted from them. I said I wanted them to prove there is a higher power because I haven't been able to find it. I couldn't live the way I had been anymore. I couldn't stand hating myself as much as I did.

I was so fed up with feeling bad about me lying and stealing for drugs, wondering how I was going to get through each day. I was just fed up with the whole life. Many times in the past, especially when I was withdrawing and the depression was so bad, I remember thinking, if I could, I would like to commit suicide. But part of me thought that if I stuck around it was bound to get worse, and I was curious. I had to see how it could get worse.

The first night there I wrote a letter to God and I said, "You know, God, if you're there you better find me in this unit because I don't know what I'm going to do from this point on. I have nothing. I tried it all and none of it's working. I've got to find a way to live." And the next day on the unit I started learning from everyone and everything. It became therapy twenty-four hours a day.

I started to learn how to be authentic. I didn't have to go in and look good anymore. I didn't want to. I felt so bad that I wanted everyone to be able to see this is how bad it's gotten.

The first three days were real difficult to adjust. They gave me a couple days to ease into the program and then, it's like—"this is what's expected. This is how we run the place and you are as important a part of this group as anyone here." It was a completely full schedule from morning until night, with no time to sit and mope.

We got up at 6:30 and had all our vital functions checked. There was meditation, then breakfast, then a lecture and then group therapy. I said, "Okay, I'm going to do it all and get my money's worth." So, for the first time in my life I was active every hour of every day. I played volleyball, ran track and rode bicycles. And I ate like a pig. All my compulsive behavior went from drugs to food immediately. I don't know how they managed. I'm sure most of our money went to buying food.

After lunch there was another group therapy, then a little break, and then at 3:30 we had story time. Each day a different person got to share his story. What her problems had been, what it had been like for him. And then we had maybe an hour to go in and do our writing.

We had dinner at five o'clock, then from six or 6:30 we'd have speakers from AA. At 7:30 there would be an AA or a CA [Cocaine Anonymous] meeting. I went to Overeaters Anonymous meetings. So everything was right there, a real cozy little place.

"Everyone is like a mirror held up to you."

To me, group therapy was the best. There's something about it that gets more out than even one-to-one therapy. You don't get to hide. But you also don't get attacked. Nobody wanted to see someone hurt. But at the same time the disease of addiction can kill us and if you're denying something, you need to have it gently brought out. Group helped me as much as anything in that treatment program. Everyone is like a mirror held up to you.

There was one guy who irked me from the day I met him. I wanted to just grab him by the throat. I got violent when he was around. But he actually liked me and had no idea I couldn't stand him. He'd come and ask me for advice and I would try to be very kind. Finally it got to the point where one day in group I attacked him. He was whining about how he does things for everyone and nobody does anything to help him. I got furious and shouted, "I am so sick and tired of listening to you. You are such a little child. Why don't you grow up for God's sake!" Afterwards the counselors in that group told me they were uncomfortable with how mercilessly I attacked this boy. He was twenty-two and I was thirty-four. He didn't stand a chance.

It was obvious that anything that prompted that kind of passionate reaction needed to be looked at. I went back to my room and I wrote and thought about why he bothered me so much. It hit me like a stone. He possessed every lousy character defect that I had and couldn't admit to. He was wallowing in the same kind of self-pity that kept me out of treatment for five years. As long as I had blamed my addiction on the whole world, I didn't have to take any action.

So I had to say to myself, "Okay, Tricia, you wasted five years. Maybe you should have been in treatment when you were twenty-nine. But you have to learn how to forgive yourself for wasting time." So I learned to forgive myself and then I started liking that guy. We're actually very good friends today. He's a nice kid.

Thirty days of treatment was a complete 180-degree turn-around. They taught me everything I needed to learn. I finally figured out I didn't have to make sure the world turned every day. I could leave things to this higher power. I had been in there about eight days and figured out *that's* what they're trying to tell me.

There is something that's more powerful. And things do happen for a reason. Sure it took me this long to get where I am. But at least I got here.

"It's all left up to something more powerful than me."

Since then it's a whole different life for me. I used to peg my self-worth on my profession. If I wasn't working in the most demanding position in a hospital then I wasn't worthwhile. I don't feel that today. I won't work as an RN, but just recently I was asked to teach classes to nurses. That's something I always wanted to do. So things are happening in their own time and I'm not running around muddling things up.

Joel and I managed somehow to stay together and grow together. He's not drinking or taking drugs. He's very calm and has a really nonalcoholic attitude towards life. He doesn't have this great need to control. We can discuss things and make decisions intelligently. We've learned to give each other what we need.

One day a few months after I left rehab I was driving along and I felt kind of nauseated. And then it hit me. I said, "Oh my God, I'm pregnant. God, please, not now! I can't take any more. I've only been sober a few months!"

Joel was totally against having a baby and we spoke about abortion. I've had abortions in the past. It was never a big deal. I had to come to terms with what I was willing to do, and for the first time in my life I realized I valued life. I had never valued it before, certainly not when I was using. If I didn't value my own life how could I value anyone else's? I couldn't even consider abortion this time. Why would anyone want to destroy a life? I told this to Joel and he said, "You've sure changed your tune."

I still have all the character defects of anyone who is an addict. I still want to be almighty. I still feel terrible when I make a mistake. But deep down I know I am a worthwhile person. And I don't wonder why I can't control this disease anymore. It's all left up to something more powerful than me.

I *have* changed. And the change feels great.

7

Marijuana
Amber's Story

Life in a Cloud of Smoke

The days when marijuana was considered a drug for hippies, dropouts and counter-culture types are definitely behind us. According to a recent NIDA survey, more than sixty million Americans have used it "in the past month."[1] Other estimates place the number of current pot users at thirty million.[2] One-third of our population now lives in states where possession of small amounts of pot has been decriminalized.[3] And the days when men were the pot smokers are also gone. In the early seventies male users outnumbered women users two to one in all age categories.[4] Today, the number of twelve- to seventeen-year-old girls reporting recent use is about the same as the number of boys.[5] One-third of young women who have ever tried marijuana say they have used it "during the past month."[6]

Smoking a joint or two, a lot of women seem to be saying, is no big deal. Sixty percent of young adult females have tried marijuana. One in ten housewives, and one in five women in professional, managerial and blue-collar jobs, have smoked pot "within the past month."[7]

But for many of the recovering women we spoke with, pot *was* a big deal. Now that the smoke has cleared, they recognize pot use as a rite of passage. One woman told us, "I thought it was okay to smoke pot. Pot was safe. But later on I didn't care. I got loaded on whatever was around."

For us, too, smoking pot was like crossing a border. It wooed us into a world of altered perceptions, heightened sensuality, new experiences of time and space and alternate lifestyles. But it did other things, too. It blunted our ambitions. It estranged us from our parents. It isolated us from friends who didn't use. It became a wall between us and normal society. People who didn't smoke now seemed square, their aspirations petty, their hard work futile, their values empty. And once this alienation had set in, there was only one way to relieve it: LSD, coke, Quaaludes.

Is this the old take-a-puff-of-marijuana-and-you'll-end-up-hooked-on-heroin school of thought? Not exactly. Very few people report using more potent drugs after smoking pot only once or twice. But *continued* marijuana use is another story. According to NIDA, ninety percent of young adults who use cocaine, hallucinogens or nonprescribed pills first smoked pot, and most of them smoked it more than ten times.[8]

Not only can pot smoking play an integral role in a female addict's slide into drug dependency, it's often the drug she is least willing to cite as part of her drug problem. Its aura of "harmlessness" can keep her smoking long after she has stopped drinking, snorting and popping pills. After all, she may reason, grass doesn't make her violent or crazed or destroy her physical well-being the way the other drugs did. But recovering women told us that holding on to pot weakened their resolve, sapped their vitality, impaired their sense of responsibility, distorted their thinking and ultimately led them back to other drugs. The reality is, no woman can walk the road of sobriety with a joint in her hand.

Alerting women, especially young women, to the dangers of marijuana is a difficult job at best, because the exaggerated scare tactics of past decades play like parodies in today's more permissive times. A few puffs on a joint is this generation's social martini. And for many, casual pot smoking may indeed be no more harmful than a glass of wine. But others aren't always so lucky. Recent research indicates that chronic use of marijuana may subtly damage parts of the brain in ways that mimic the effects of aging.[9] Marijuana is also believed to suppress that part of the immune system that plays a role in resisting viral infection and cancer.[10] Recent studies show that pot can cause panic attacks and an intense fear of leaving one's home. In some cases, these fearful episodes can continue long after the user has stopped smoking.[11] A 1987 study also suggested that pot may cause or activate schizophrenia.[12] And there is compelling evidence to suggest that marijuana can affect the development of an unborn child.[13] Pot's acceptability, then, is not testimony to its relative harmlessness; it is the hallmark of its insidiousness.

Prevailing wisdom has it that marijuana is not addictive. But those who have tried it more than ten times are not liable to give it up. And anyone who has seen a woman light up a joint in the early morning because she "can't start the day without a puff" knows that pot can trigger obsessive dependency as surely as any other drug.

In the story that follows, we see one woman's experience of how pot smoking started casually, then became the center of her life.

Amber's story also offers us a glimpse into an intriguing phenomenon. In some families in which a teen is abusing alcohol or drugs, it is not uncommon for the parents to say, "The kid didn't learn that behavior at home." Not only do they themselves not use drugs, they sincerely insist, but they've never even been tipsy. It often turns out that these parents were themselves raised in alcoholic homes. As adults they have been determined not to repeat the mistakes of their parents, or even to talk about them. All the fear, anger, and emotional charge around alcohol and drugs go underground; the ACA issues seem to have skipped a generation. In fact, they merely tiptoed through it. As long as these issues are unresolved and untreated, they remain potent and disturbing influences in the family system.

*   *   *

Amber's Story

*We went to interview Amber on the campus of a
university where she is getting an advanced degree in
psychology. She is a slim, delicate woman with shoulder-
length brown hair. Although she is in her late twenties,
she has the vibrancy of a teenager. At the time we met,
Amber had been clean and sober for six months.*

What really stands out about my whole life is that I lived a lie. I was
the strong one in my family. Whenever things got bad, I was the one
who took care of things. I was like a little mother, always acting as
if I didn't have any needs of my own and everything was fine. But
on the inside I was just falling apart and there was no one I could
talk to. There was no one.

I didn't sleep well and I hated eating. Every day I had these
horrible anxiety attacks. I had been having them since I was nine,
when my parents got divorced. I was really torn up by that. I used
to hide in the bushes, crying and praying to God to please let my
parents get back together, and I'd do anything, sacrifice anything. I
thought that if I took my life for my family they would be okay. At
age nine I thought about and made half-hearted attempts at killing
myself. I was so depressed.

The first time I ever felt relieved was when I was fourteen and
first took drugs. That was a turning point for me.

"Drugs were a liberation."

I started out by smoking pot with a couple of friends at a music
festival. I went crazy on it. I wanted to get as out of it as I could
get. Pot gave me a feeling of power. The outside world couldn't get
to me anymore. People couldn't get to me anymore. I wasn't under
their thumbs anymore. That was the only way I could take my life
back.

To me smoking marijuana was seeing the world in a whole new way. It was like I was free, almost omnipotent. The world was at my feet and all the everyday, boring, mundane things were so interesting. Everything took on a whole new meaning. I had this power. I was above it all. I couldn't be touched. I was transformed into a new level where things couldn't bring me down.

Drugs were a liberation; a wonderful, grand liberation. From the moment I started using I didn't have those nightly paranoid anxiety attacks anymore. I felt like I got along better in the world, like I fit in. And I didn't have to deal with parents.

Both my parents came from alcoholic homes. My dad was real unfeeling, almost a kind of cruel person. My mom focused all her attention on me. She was obsessive about me throughout my childhood. We were so close that there were almost no boundaries between us. Taking drugs put a wedge between me and my mom. A nice big wedge. I remember Christmas time when I was fourteen; I passed out on the table from some kind of downer. My mom just thought I was kind of tired.

Almost immediately after discovering pot I started doing uppers, downers, whatever my friends could get their hands on. I never turned anything down. I think if someone had walked up to me and offered to shoot heroin into my arm I would probably have said yes. By the time I was seventeen I was doing LSD about once a week but I was having so many bad trips that I had to stop. I didn't even smoke dope or drink or anything for about a year.

But pot was always the thing I went back to, so eventually I started smoking again. I don't think I ever had to buy it at that time. I just used it when it was around. I'd get it from friends or from my older brother. I used to ditch class and smoke with him. I tried speed, white crosses, and coke for a while but I got real paranoid. That scared me and I had to stop.

"It wasn't like using a drug."

When I turned eighteen I moved in with a man. He was a real pothead, loaded all the time. That's when I started smoking daily. It was there and he did it and we were together so I would just do it. I could tell that he needed it, but I didn't feel that I needed it at all. I lived with him for about six and a half years and most of that time we were smoking daily.

We bought a house together with a second bedroom which had two pads under the carpet and we put pillows down on the floor and we had the stereo in there and we called it the music room. We'd go in there, turn the stereo up, get out the dope and sit on the floor on the pillows and pass the dope back and forth.

It was so much a part of everyday life that it wasn't like using a drug. It was just part of what I did. And it made everything nice. It relaxed me. It took away my problems. I didn't think I had problems. It somehow made me feel at peace. It had a real nice euphoric effect on me. It was a big part of how I related to him.

In the early seventies through the late seventies we grew our own. We had this big plot out in the back yard, oh, about the size of this room. It was covered over with plastic. We'd plant it and for the most part he'd take care of it. Then we'd hang it up and dry it. That gave us way more than we needed. We didn't sell it. We just used it and gave it away.

I was drinking maybe once or twice a month and not using other drugs, so the only thing I was doing as a habit was smoking dope. I was working part-time as a bookkeeper and getting my bachelor's degree in psychology. A few times I went to work loaded, but it interfered so badly I didn't do it very often.

When my boyfriend and I broke up I got in with a different crowd of people and started drinking a lot more because we were going out to bars all the time. My pot consumption went way down, to about once a week. Then a couple of years later I got into my next serious relationship with a guy at work who was a real pothead.

"We really got into sex."

With the first guy we just got mellow together. In this second relationship we combined alcohol and pot and got out of it all the time, to the point where we were totally irresponsible. We never washed a dish, never cleaned up, never did anything we were supposed to do. We just got wasted.

I never missed work because of pot or alcohol but I wasn't conscientious and lots of times I'd go in really late. My boyfriend was more of a periodic. He would go for a spell not using anything, turning into Mr. Responsible for a little while, but I always wanted to use, all the time. That was all I wanted to do—stay ripped. So I was always kind of pulling him back into it, 'cause he was kind of susceptible anyway.

I had gotten very crazy. I'd go through a whole personality change. Pot would energize me and I'd start bouncing off the walls, saying things that were real bizarre. I just got real crazy and loud and hyper. It wasn't relaxing anymore at all.

We were always flashing between two extremes, either having sex on cloud nine or in the middle of a horrible gut-wrenching fight. I started having blackouts sometimes, because when we fought I'd start drinking more. We were together for two years and the whole time was up and down, up and down. Nothing was ever even and I liked that. I liked the extremes. He didn't. He got tired of it and eventually we broke up.

Then my drug use changed again; it got heavier. I started smoking dope and drinking with girlfriends just about every night.

I decided that any scruple I could drop I was all the better for dropping. I thought I was all hung up from my really moral upbringing. I didn't want all that stuff. I decided—f— men. I'm just going to go have a good time and not get committed to anyone.

Every night, the second we got off work, my best friend and I got into the car where we had a joint rolled and passed it back and forth. After we got loaded we went to a bar and drank.

She was a real dope fiend. I was very attracted to people who used marijuana all the time. And when I was with them I used it all the time. It sounds like I'm blaming everybody else. Maybe I am.

"My relationships were totally centered around drugs."

By this time, I was buying my pot. It was mostly cheap stuff 'cause I couldn't afford the good stuff. I remember thinking that buying was a real symptom of being an addict.

I had all these different stashes—one in my car, one in my purse, one I kept at home, then a backup one at home. I'd take a little stash over to a friend's house as if it was all I had. But I'd make sure that I had stuff hidden away that they didn't know about so we could freely use what I had out and I wouldn't have to worry about them using it all up. Later when I threw out all my stuff, I was surprised to find five or six different places where I had stuffed it away.

Then, for about a year, I got involved with two men at the same time. One of them travelled a lot so I saw him maybe two or three times a month and the other one I saw two or three times a week. The one who travelled was an alcoholic. We drank and sometimes smoked together. But I was always disappointed that he didn't like to smoke more. The other one would smoke anytime and he also drank. My relationships with these men were totally centered around using drugs and alcohol. That's what we did together, usually at their houses because I took such terrible care of my own house I couldn't let anyone near it.

I'd bring dope with me and we'd start smoking and drinking as soon as I got there. And then we'd have sex. I loved sex with marijuana. I used to feel like I was in heaven—well, better than heaven.

"I had no intention of not smoking dope anymore."

The first time I thought I had a problem was a year ago last month. I was in a new job, real stressed out at work, and I was using marijuana and alcohol every day. I'd get off work and I'd get into the parking lot and I couldn't wait to get the joint in my mouth. If for some reason I had to delay that for an hour, I would be climbing walls. I wanted to get that joint in my mouth and get to a bar and get a drink.

One guy I'd been seeing was worried about how much I depended on pot and booze. So over the following several months I started thinking more about my alcohol use. Around that time I found ACA [Adult Children of Alcoholics] for the first time. And I learned a little bit about what addiction was and when I heard that, I recognized that I had a problem.

The speaker talked about how ACAs have a much higher rate of alcoholism, that they drink—and this is true for drug use, too— because they had something missing as a child. So if you were a very responsible child, you had an overdeveloped sense of responsibility but you never learned how to relax, have fun, and play or socialize, and you use the drug or the alcohol to do that for you, to fill in what was missing. Or if you were a people-pleaser like I was, then you use the drugs and the alcohol to get to a point where you can say, "F— you, I don't care what you think." So, you use the drugs and alcohol to make you feel like a whole person. And that's what I did. When I used either marijuana or alcohol I felt like I could be myself, and when I wasn't using it, I couldn't. I was at the mercy of all these people who had all these expectations and I was worried about what they thought of me. I think that has to do partly with being a woman, too—this thing about having to meet other people's needs all the time. That was what I was relieved of when I smoked dope and drank booze. I stopped drinking in October and started going to AA. But I had no intentions of not smoking dope anymore.

At AA meetings I heard people talking about how they had to give up marijuana. I didn't want to give it up. I remember thinking, "What am I going to have to live for?" I mean, that's how I felt about it. All my important relationships had been built around dope. All the times I could think of when life was worth living was when I was smoking dope.

There was this big meeting that had about two hundred people and most of them were NA people. And I was sitting in that meeting feeling like I wanted to smoke some dope. I was sitting way at the back. I was as far away from the leader as you could get but I was the first person he called on. And I shared at this meeting how I felt about dope. And the whole room started laughing.

Afterwards, a bunch of people came up to me. "You're not going to get the benefits of the program if you continue to use," one woman said. "And it's going to keep you one step closer to going back into the drinking. A lot of people start drinking again because they're doing other drugs." And I believed her. I felt, "These people all can't be wrong. They didn't want to give it up any more than I do. If they could do it, I can do it."

"It's like I'm a kid again."

At first it was a shock getting sober. I felt awful. I didn't know that's what crashing was like, having to go through the bad parts without fixing it. I was used to fixing myself right away, putting a joint in my mouth and making all the feelings go away. I didn't wait to see what was going to happen the next minute, much less the next week. It's not always easy doing it this way and there are times, in the last six months, when I wonder, "Why in the hell did I ever give up smoking dope?"

I have to remind myself about the misery I used to feel between joints. I used to have a feeling in my gut that something was very, very wrong, something so wrong with me that I'm going to die from it. I used to feel like I was rotting, just rotting inside. And I don't have that anymore.

I got this new job. I have the first serious relationship I've been in for a while. And I'm learning how to do things. I feel like I'm starting over again. It's like I'm a kid again. I'm learning how to be a person without drugs. You know, that's what it feels like. And learning how to have friends and be able to have fun with them. I'm learning how to have a boyfriend. I never had a boyfriend where the central part of it wasn't drugs.

I had one experience that I've never had before in my life and I know it was related to being clean and sober. I was standing in the shower and I felt like it was a gift to be alive. I had never had that feeling before in my life.

I'm just at the first step of everything but I see what can happen. I've seen people who have lost everything by the time they stop drinking and using, people who were miserable and half-dead. And I've seen them sober, enjoying life and appreciating life. I've seen that enough that I believe it. I believe that can happen to me. And that's what kind of keeps me going. At this point it's mostly based on hope. I still am mostly going on hope.

8

Cocaine
Nanci's Story

The Party's Over

Cocaine isn't just a man's problem anymore. Since 1983 the number of women calling 800-COCAINE, the national cocaine helpline, has risen eighteen percent. Women now account for nearly half of all calls.[1]

Cocaine isn't just for jet setters anymore. According to the National Institute on Drug Abuse (NIDA), twenty-two million Americans have tried cocaine, five million are regular users and two million are dependent on the drug. Other researchers place the numbers of regular users at *twenty-four* million.[2]

Cocaine can't be considered just fun anymore. It's a killer. Laboratory animals given unlimited access to cocaine killed themselves at nearly three times the rate of those given access to heroin.[3] NIDA now calls cocaine one of the most powerfully addictive substances known. Each year, as many as ten thousand women wind up in hospital emergency rooms because of cocaine. It is a factor in more than ten percent of female drug fatalities.[4]

Cocaine is everywhere. It is in our businesses, our homes, our playing fields and our schools. Twice as many high school seniors now try it as did ten years ago, and half of all seniors admit that cocaine is readily available to them.[5]

Use of cocaine is increasing more rapidly than any other mood-changing substance. The number of people who have tried cocaine has doubled in the past five years, and the number of people who have tried it "recently" has tripled. By 1985, every single day, five thousand people were trying cocaine for the first time.[6]

Women start using cocaine at an earlier age and use larger quantities than men. At one treatment center, women who had bought their own cocaine had spent five hundred to one thousand dollars a week on it, twice as much money on it as men did.[7]

Because cocaine gives the dangerous illusion of peak-functioning, it is increasingly becoming the drug of today's overachieving women. A 1985 *New York Times* article reported that its use is four times greater among professional and working women than among women who work in the home.[8]

And cocaine is as welcome in the bedroom as in the boardroom. "Guys used to bring us flowers," said one woman, "now they bring us cocaine." In a 1985 survey of 800-COCAINE contacts, eighty-seven percent of the women had been introduced to the drug by men and sixty-five percent were still receiving it as a gift from men.[9]

Women are finding out what men have known for years: cocaine adds spice to their sex lives, relaxes their inhibitions and heightens their sensations. But in the long run, as surely as it causes impotence in men, cocaine interferes with a woman's sexual satisfaction and can make her nonorgasmic.[10]

And while it is an old story that some women turn to prostitution to support their heroin habits, cocaine has given rise to a new phenomenon: "coke whores"—women who have sex not for cash, or even pleasure, but for their drug. As one doctor put it, "To be able to afford cocaine, you either have to be rich or cunning."[11]

Coke is the "recreational drug" of the eighties, but even so-called recreational doses can be deadly. Coke users continue to have an increased risk of heart failure long after they stop taking even moderate amounts of the drug. Cokers in their twenties and thirties are suffering heart attacks after taking relatively small doses of cocaine.[12] And chronic use of "safe" doses makes the user more susceptible to brain seizures which can lead to death.[13] At high-dose use, cocaine produces psychosis, a state of mind characterized by paranoia and delusions.[14]

For women of child-bearing age, cocaine can be devastating. When used during pregnancy it increases the risk of miscarriages. In one study, thirty-eight percent of cocaine-using woman suffered spontaneous abortions.[15] Stillborns and fetal deaths are twice as likely to be caused by cocaine as by any other drug.[16] And there is growing evidence of a fetal cocaine syndrome. Babies born of cocaine-using mothers can suffer congenital abnormalities and may have suffered minor strokes because of changes in the mother's blood pressure. As newborns they display visual problems, erratic and unresponsive behavior, and are far more difficult to comfort than normal babies.[17]

The jolt of euphoria that follows a dose of cocaine lasts at most about an hour. Staying high means taking more coke, or some speed. A survey of people calling a cocaine hotline revealed that seventy percent had binged out on coke—used it continuously for twenty-four hours or more.[18]

But eventually even superwoman comes down, and many women try to counter cocaine's long-range downside—depression, insomnia, irritability, digestive disorders, dangerous weight loss, malnutrition, rapid heartbeat, paranoia, and hallucinations such as "cocaine bugs"—with other drugs. We've yet to meet a woman who abused cocaine who didn't also wind up using large doses of tranquilizers or alcohol to counteract coke jitters.

It's impossible to exaggerate the hold cocaine had on our own lives. It started as a party—lots of people, lots of laughter, a couple of lines on a fancy mirror and a sterling silver straw. It ended with furtive, solitary snorts in the nearest bathroom every fifteen or twenty minutes. We were a couple of wrecks, but in our own minds we were operating at the peak of efficiency. In four years our daily doses had grown from two lines to half a gram each. We lived under constant emotional duress and faced financial ruin. Then, seven years ago, on our last cocaine Christmas, as our children opened their presents, we sat grinding our teeth, praying for the day to be over, and we had a glimpse of the cold emptiness at the core of cocaine living.

Most people who regularly take cocaine toot it, and an increasing number smoke it as freebase in the form called crack. Only a comparative few seem to mainline it regularly, but a recent NIDA survey found that eighty percent of cocaine users had experimented with intravenous injection.[19] IV drug use is considered by some authorities the route by which AIDS will cross over from the high risk population into mainstream society. Cocaine use, then, may soon prove to be the biggest factor of all in the spread of AIDS.

The two stories that follow focus on the two most common ways of taking cocaine: tooting it and smoking crack.

* * *

Nanci's Story

*We interviewed Nanci at her Victorian-style house in a
small beach community south of L.A., where she lives
with her husband and two-year-old son. Nanci is a small
and shapely woman in her early twenties. She wears her
blonde hair cut short. At the time of this interview,
Nanci had been clean and sober six months.*

I was sixteen the first time I had cocaine. I had gone to Hawaii with
my family and we were coming back on a first class flight. I had
really beautiful boobs. I was wearing a peach blouse with a criss-
cross front and tight white pants on my tanned skin. Sitting across
the aisle from us was the model in the [cigarette brand] ads and he
was gorgeous. He was sitting with some members of [well-known
rock band]. My father said, "Look at those animals," but I thought,
"Wow, this is it!" When they went up to the lounge, I followed
them. My father asked, "Where are you going?" and I said I was
going upstairs so I'd feel less airsick. I sat with the cigarette man
and the band and they asked me if I would like to smoke a joint
and I said yes. They had cocaine and they gave me my first line and
it was wonderful. I thought, "How glamorous." Then the rock star
asked me if I knew how they did it on airplanes. I said no, how did
they do it on airplanes and he asked, "Would you like to go to the
bathroom?" I said I didn't have to go. That's how naive I was.

    I grew up in a huge mansion in Hong Kong where we were
known as one of the richest families. My grandfather had started an
import-export company and when he died my father took it over. I
lived there till I was sixteen and a half years old.

    I was a wild, rebellious child, always wanting to be the leader
of the group. I never let anyone see that I was scared. When I was
ten I started smoking cigarettes, then opiated pot when I was
thirteen. They took a stick of dope and dipped it in opium. So I was
brought into the opiates as a kid and I loved it.

    I only saw my father once in a while. My mother was involved
in bazaars, charity, and played a lot of golf. And she was always

knitting. You ever try to talk to your mother about something and she's sitting there knitting? And when she doesn't like something you're saying, she knits real hard. That's how I was loved. And I got coldness from my father. See, my father was my god, but he never gave me any love. I've never met any woman cokehead who had a loving and wonderful relationship with her father.

When I came to the United States at sixteen and got off the plane, my face was green and I was vomiting. I had lost my voice. I was really sick. The doctors told me I had walking pneumonia and put me in bed for three weeks. I know today that I was in full-blown withdrawal from opium.

My parents bought this beautiful multimillion-dollar house in California overlooking the ocean. I went to school in a very snobby, very wealthy area—it was horrendous. Nobody liked me. I talked different, I looked different, I felt different, I was different. But I did know how to smoke cigarettes and I did know what good dope was.

It took me a couple of weeks to find *the* ladies' bathroom in school, but I found it. They were all sitting there drinking and smoking grass and I walked in and got loaded with them. I instantly had friends. But the dope, after Southeast Asia, would not get me high. It wouldn't do it.

"I think they raped me but I don't remember."

There was a guy I knew who had a chemist friend in San Francisco who made MDA [a synthetic drug related to mescaline and amphetamine]. The first time I did it I loved it. It did more for me than anything had ever done for me—my father, my mother, a boyfriend, a joint—anything. It was wonderful. So I said, "Look. You give me a lot of it, I'll sell it for you and make some money for you." He goes, "Here, take it." So I started dealing MDA and I was on MDA for a year and a half straight. No stopping. Every day. In the morning I'd buy a can of Dr. Pepper at a convenience store. I'd take a capful out of my little MDA bottle and I'd go. I went to school on it. I went to work on it. I was always on acid, too, and it was very important in my life right then. It just got me out. I could go to never-never land on acid, whereas cocaine made my mind work, it made me dwell on situations and it became too intense.

Whenever I did cocaine at that time in my life, I had to have LSD or some kind of downer because I would get too crazy.

I don't remember how it all came up about this time but my parents had cut me off financially and I wasn't living at home. They had said, "You're out." I'm not really sure what happened the next two years, but I got into a lot of trouble. One weekend I overdosed on thirty-two hits of LSD. I don't remember who found me. I was a blackout user who would black out and pass out. People always had to tell me what happened to me. All I remember is my mother and father flipping out at some hospital.

But the biggest thing I remember was, when I was seventeen, I took a lot of Quaaludes, drank a whole bunch of alcohol, smoked some dope, and jumped off a cliff. I didn't want to live anymore. There was a cement sidewalk that went along the beach with rocks here and there and a little tiny patch of sand. I missed the sidewalk, I missed the rocks. I landed in the little bump of sand. I lay there, thinking I would die. All I remember was some guys finding me and putting me in a van. I think they raped me but I don't remember. I woke up on the beach with my clothing ripped.

I didn't have any money so, by this time, I was doing cocaine only when someone offered it to me. Coke dealers didn't want to mess with me because I was messing with other drugs and I was a risk. I was constantly getting picked up by the police: not arrested, just picked up for being on the street. They knew me. They knew I had drugs. They knew I was dealing. They also played golf with my father. So it all worked out.

Then came the last straw for my parents. I had gone back to living with them but I had disappeared for about three days and came home still on acid. My mother went through my purse and found a lot of drugs. A little bit of this, a little bit of that. She took me down to the police station at like ten o'clock at night and they had it analyzed and told her, "We're going to have to do something about this," and she said, "No, I can't turn in my own daughter."

The next night I dropped off some MDA and I had no way to get home so I hitchhiked. This man gave me a ride and told me I was a stupid little girl. That's all I remember. I walked into my parents' house and said, "I want help." And my parents said, "Okay, you can come to Montana where we're going for the summer. We'll buy you a horse. Take care of you. Give you everything you want if you just stay off of drugs.''

I said, ''You got it. I'm going.'' I went, but I had my ounce of dope, my pills and a jar of hash oil. So I was stocked for at least a month. I ended up staying there the whole year. I smoked pot and I drank in the bars and I got in a lot of trouble but my parents could accept it because it was nothing like what I had done before.

Then I met Fred. He was thirty-two and I was seventeen years old. I felt like hot sh—. We got married.

"Cocaine allowed me to be erotic."

In 1980 or '81, Fred and I moved in with my sister and brother-in-law and we all had a lot of money and that's when I started getting heavily into cocaine. I was getting three thousand dollars every Christmas from my grandmother, as interest payments on the trust. We chipped in for an ounce of cocaine. It was the most exciting moment of my life. All that beautiful powder. We got our big beautiful wine glasses and we got beautiful champagne. I got all dressed up and I can remember sitting there and saying ''Oh, darling—'' I don't remember what I was wearing, but I know it was flamboyant and I know I had a lot of makeup on, and I know I was having an orgasm from the cocaine. I just knew everything was fine. I didn't need you. You didn't need me. But come on over here baby and I don't care who you are or what you look like. Get over here!

I could have sex. Wow. Sex was wonderful on cocaine, unbelievable. I mean, I had never been into oral sex. On cocaine, put it all over me. Put it all over you. Cocaine allowed me to be erotic and wear black negligees. It allowed me to be anyone I wanted to be. I could walk into a bar with no bra on, down to here in a size three pair of pants and shake my a—. On cocaine I had no such thing as shame or guilt. I never knew how to feel. I took the drug and what the drug did, I felt.

At that point the cocaine was every day. Every moment. Wake up with coffee and with cocaine and get into how we're going to fix the world and sit there and analyze feelings and talk about things you don't know. It was very wonderful.

Friends had found out we had coke and the pile got smaller. People weren't doing what they should have been doing in this very small house. Beer bottles everywhere, beautiful furniture getting ruined. We weren't sleeping or eating. My sister thought I wanted to sleep with her husband and she flipped out. She smashed all her beautiful china on the floor and kicked us out. Her husband left. This is what cocaine did for us in a week. The cocaine was down to maybe three grams. One for me. One for you. And we'll split the other and sell it.

We moved and bought an eight-baller [an eighth of an ounce] just to get rolling. We didn't have any money but it was okay. We just bought small amounts and that did it. We would buy like a gram or two grams and it was nice. Fred wasn't really into cocaine. He was into the drinking.

"I wanted glamor. I wanted excitement."

I got a job in a hotel. And now we're talking about Nanci getting off work at 3 A.M., whiff some coke, go out drinking, partying or whatever, come home, whiff some more coke, and have sex. It got real boring.

Well, our money started to run out again. So the next alternative was crank: crystal Methedrine. I mean, we're talking about burning your nose and throwing up blood. Your eyes are . . . [sound of pain]! You can't move. This happened within a three-month period and I was going insane. So I quit my job. I knew it was the job. I threw my pencil at the boss and said, "F— you, go to hell." I just took black beauties for about three weeks while I went looking for a new job.

I got a job in a car rental place in Los Angeles and I thought, "I'll meet some great people who do a lot of drugs and I'll find a coke dealer." That was the main thing, because I had burned out all my connections by calling them at three or four in the morning. Then I found out, Monday after the Fourth of July, that I was three and a half months pregnant. Which meant for the first three months I had been doing all these drugs—black beauties, mushrooms—all of it. I told the doctor I had done a few drugs. He asked me what and I told him it was none of his business. I thought he was going to turn me in.

Anyway, I stopped doing drugs and got very ill. I couldn't go to work. I started hemorrhaging and throwing up constantly, and I went into kidney failure. The doctor said, "No one can be this sick from just pregnancy. You must be low on estrogen and progesterone." It wasn't progesterone. It wasn't estrogen. I was withdrawing from tremendous amounts of drugs.

I almost lost the baby. They wanted to abort him at six months. They prepared us in a roundabout way that it would be deformed. All I wanted to know when that baby was born was—was he okay? Does he have ten fingers, ten toes, two this, two that? And he was a healthy, beautiful, seven-pound, fifteen-ounce boy.

There was occasional drinking, smoking and a little coke until Timmy was a year old. I was getting ten thousand dollars every six months. I was in seventh heaven. The summer of 1982—where was I?—my God, I can't even remember. Timmy's first Christmas I was loaded and hung over. By Timmy's first birthday in 1983, I realized that being a mother was not going to make me happy.

A month later, on my twenty-first birthday, I bought as much cocaine as I could. I bought as much champagne and pot as I could. I had a punk party. You had to come in punk and if you didn't have any coke, don't come. That was what the invitation said. We had strippers. Everybody put their coke on the table and we whiffed all night long.

By June my habit was up to at least two or three grams a week so Timmy was not getting a lot of good care. I would sedate him. I had cough syrup from the doctor and, when I couldn't wake up in the morning, "Here, take some cough syrup." My marriage no longer meant anything. And my child no longer meant anything to me. I wanted glamor. I wanted excitement. I didn't want to be a mother anymore, and I sure as hell didn't want to be a wife.

I was just obnoxious. My girlfriends didn't want to hang around with me anymore. I was falling down drunk. In two weeks I spent twelve hundred dollars. Fred said to me, "Where did it go?" And I said, "It was my money, a— hole. F— you and die."

"His name was Christopher and he looked like Billy Idol."

Then I decided I was going to straighten up my life. I jogged and started to feel good. For three weeks I stopped all cocaine. I was just taking speed, smoking and drinking champagne. I tried to get my marriage going with Fred and was trying to be a good mother, going to Disneyland, buying all kinds of toys and making fabulous dinners that no one even ate. I enrolled in hotel/motel management school.

Then a girlfriend of mine showed up. She was dealing a lot of coke and we started getting loaded together. One night we were both depressed and decided we're going to the Hilton Hotel where we could drink and no men would harass us. We got drunk and said, "F— it—let's go to a bar and have some good times." We walked into the Brown Steer and that's were I met my destruction. A blond-haired man walked up and asked me to dance. His name was Christopher and he looked like Billy Idol. I said, "Oh yes, I'd love to dance." I had dressed up very glamorously in a three hundred dollar outfit and my diamonds and a really punk hairdo. I looked good. The cocaine made me think I was Farrah Fawcett punked out.

He said, "Well, what do you do?" I said, "What do you mean?" He said, "Well, I got a little cola." I go, "What?" "You do cola, don't you?" "Is it that white stuff?" He said, "You've never done cola, you've never done blow?" I said, "Oh I think I tried it once. I think it was in Greece." And he goes, "Shall we go do some lines?" I said, "Oh sure." He looks at my girlfriend and says, "I don't have enough for her." I said, "Lisa, f— off. We'll be right back. I got a live one." We go in the head and do a couple of lines. It was sh—ty coke. I said, "Well darling, it's time for me to leave." And he said, "Call me, call me."

I called him and we met Wednesday night. We screwed in the car. And he said, "God, I've never met a girl that has done this to me before. It usually takes some wining and dining." And I said, "Honey, you *will* do the wining and dining." There was no coke that night but he knew where to get some. I let on that I wanted the connection. And he introduced me.

I met the connection Friday night at Munchums. I was all dressed up in a grey cashmere sweater, my diamonds and snakeskin high heels. The dealer was a scrawny Jewish man who loved me. Here I was, a glamorous woman with plenty of money who could pay cash for her grams when everybody else wanted to be fronted. We started buying from him that night, and every night we'd come back three and four times a night. This would start out about eight o'clock and by six in the morning we were finally getting our last gram. It got to the point where I was doing about an ounce a week.

Nobody knew. I had three coke dealers and I would hit a different one each time. I didn't want anyone to know I was a cokehead.

I had to hide the coke. I had three or four hiding places. I had one under the bed, one in my drawer and one in the bathroom. If I had to go to the bathroom, like, I didn't constantly run upstairs. I was very good at what I did. Nobody knew. Nobody. I would whiff half a gram at a time, then I'd be okay for an hour. Even Fred didn't know how bad it had gotten.

I would just whiff and whiff and whiff, clean the house, do this and do that and I thought it was really glamorous. I was down to 108 pounds, to a size three pants. I weigh 120 pounds, 125 at my best. I wasn't eating.

"This is what I wanted—a house full of drug addicts."

At noon, no matter what, there were the soap operas. Cocaine and soap operas were wonderful. I had this beautiful antique mirror and I always had champagne with me. I used to sit here in this exact spot and I'd chop, and I'd chop, and I'd chop, and I'd chop. Once someone timed me and said it took me thirty-five minutes to chop my coke. I had to have it fine so it wouldn't get caught in my nose. It always upset me the way people used to pick their noses and then eat it because there was coke in it.

Fred was always flaming drunk at the time. I wanted him out of the house. I wanted Christopher to come over and sleep with me in my house. I wanted to walk into a bar in nice clothes, a pocket full of cocaine and a man who made the other women look at me and made me feel okay. So I kicked Fred out of the house. Timmy stayed with me.

When I was with Christopher I bought all the drugs and things. That was the deal. He was paid for. He did what I wanted him to do. We'd find a party or go to a bar, hang out, and end up back here. Nanci's became the after-hours hangout. I'd have thirty, forty people here. A lot of my jewels got stolen. I had people passed out and throwing up in my house. I had a two-year-old who was not getting fed and a sixteen-year-old babysitter who was whiffing coke, smoking dope, and drinking with me.

I had it made. This is what I wanted—a house full of drug addicts and alcoholics to party with me, accept me, and think I had the baddest life of all. That was what I wanted and I found it. And after a while I didn't want it, so we condensed it down to six or seven of us. We'd sit here in this room, smoke a tremendous amount of pot, drink two or three cases of beer, a bottle of tequila, and somebody always had an eight ball.

One beautiful summer day at six in the morning we drove down to South Laguna. We climbed down the cliff and we all made love on the beach and it was great. That's what I wanted to do. You know. That's what I wanted. My one ultimate in life was to be with a man I sexually adored and to be glamorous, spectacular, and make love on the beach. That was my goal in life. I cried, because I knew my life was over and it was time to kill myself. See, my kid no longer meant anything to me. Money didn't. Christopher didn't anymore. What was left to live for?

A few nights later I went over to his house crying, insane. I told him private investigators were after me. I called the police to get restraining orders on Fred and told them somebody's got to help me because there are three unmarked cars after me, they've got a private investigator on me, and they're going to kill me.

Christopher looked at me and said, "Let's do a line and then we'll talk about it." We got f—ed up that night. I went home and those cars were there. Oh my God, those cars. Where's Timmy? I couldn't remember where Timmy was. Who has Timmy? Someone stole my son. He's gone. I had taken him to his f—ing father's house. It was my mind that was gone.

"I had half an ounce of cocaine in my bra."

I decided I needed a vacation. I'll go visit this guy I met, Mark, who lives in Washington. I call him and he tells me, "Great. Bring some coke." I figured I'd buy half an ounce. But this time I got smart: I'm going to go to the big guys to buy my coke. I can do that. I'm big enough. I've got enough money. I had met one of them, just by accident, but he didn't want to deal with me. He had heard about me.

My dealer said, "You'll have to go through me." "No, I'm not going through a middle man. I want the big man." He said, "Nanci, you're insane. You are f—ing with little sh—. You want to buy a pound, you invite the big guy up." I wouldn't give him my money. So he finally gives in and these two other f—ers come to my house and I'm scared. I mean these guys have not been out on the streets in three months. Their faces are white, their eyes are sunken in and they look like they're f—ing going to die or kill. But I get my half ounce.

I start chopping up all my coke. I'm getting ready, I'm packing. I had about twelve hundred bucks cash on me and all this stuff— some here, some there, coming out of everywhere. I was a f—ing drug bank. My girlfriend comes over to drive me to the airport and we really get f—ed up. We whiffed probably about four grams in a matter of four hours so she took me to someone's house where we could get some Valiums and soapers [Quaaludes] to calm me down and have a couple of drinks. Just before we left the guy brought out a base pipe so we based for an hour. My conscience was telling me I could not leave my son for a week. My life was f—ed. I'm falling apart. I looked terrible. My girlfriend said, "What are you doing? Stop pulling your hair out. Stop it, Nanci!"

On the plane I was sweating. And the guy next to me goes, "Are you all right?" I said, "I got a touch of the flu." The plane took off and I thought I was going to throw up. I went into the bathroom, took some more coke and popped six or seven Valiums. It calmed me right down and I had a bloody mary and the guy started talking—kind of a nerd from nowhere. And I go, "Well, what do you do for a living?" He answered, "I'm a customs investigator." My heart dropped. I had half an ounce of cocaine in my bra, a quarter on this tit and a quarter on that tit, so it wouldn't look uneven. I had so many drugs on me that I just said, "Oh." And after that I don't remember anything else.

I remember getting off the plane and basically looking at Mark and saying, "I'm really f—ed up." I woke up two days later. A lot of the cocaine was gone. Not all of it. They did leave me a quarter of an ounce. They f—ing knew they better because when I woke up, I was going to require massive amounts of cocaine.

Mark had a girlfriend there and he wasn't willing to give her up even for just a week. So there was constant fighting between us. I got really drunk and threw an ashtray at some guy in a bar and hit him in the head and then I dumped all these drinks on Mark and his girlfriend. He told me it was time for me to go. And I left.

"I wanted one last time."

When I came back, I went to Fred and said, "Look I want to go to Montana. I want to get back together and I want this all to end. I'm not going to ever use cocaine again." That weekend I had my most horrendous usage.

I went out and got really f—ed up, mainly on alcohol, and I cannot handle alcohol without cocaine. I just throw up. So I bought some coke and stayed up all by myself. I loved it and it was hell. Saturday night I was with a guy and all of his friends and we got an eight ball. A good friend of mine was doing some PCP so I had a couple of toots, and that kind of got things going. I had only whiffed maybe two grams that day. I put a whole gram of coke on my mirror, chopped it all up, drew one enormous line, got my straw and I went [sound of snorting]. I felt my heart and said, "I've done it. I've got the ultimate high." I just lay there. I knew I was dying. My body shook. I said, "This is it, this is it." People were looking at me going, "What the f— are you doing?" "Nanci's dying," I thought, "and it's great."

They sat me up in a corner, but they wouldn't take me to the hospital. We were too loaded. They thought if they took me in we'd all been arrested. Today we know that's not true. I took a bunch of Valium that night and drank some tequila and then I was miserable. I had now been taking quite a few Valium to calm my nerves. Everything was flipping me out. I couldn't handle it.

Timmy came downstairs when I was flipping out and I yelled at him, "Get the hell away from me." My son used to stand in front of the walls and hit them and say "I hate you, I hate you." He didn't know what he hated, he just hated life. He was a violent child. He was really scared. That morning I heard a crash and it was him. He was in the icebox getting something to eat—he was hungry. And I beat the s— out of him. I didn't put any marks on him but I scared him—I shook him, I hit him, and that was enough.

Fred had gone to my parents and told them I had all these problems with cocaine. My parents summoned a meeting and they did an intervention on me. I told them I could handle drugs, that Fred was trying to manipulate me, trying to get me back in his life. Then my father said, "I'm going to physically cut you off—no more money. Why don't you go to one meeting at the hospital?" "Okay, I'll go." I walked in there, sat down and thought, "What the f— am I doing here?"

But I heard something. I heard you don't ever have to feel this way again. And I heard some cocaine death stories.

That night was Christopher's birthday and I wanted one last toot. I knew I had to have coke. So Christopher showed up and we're all tooting and he looked at me and said, "You're looking good." Thank God somebody liked me still. I looked like hell. There's a picture of myself from those days. My eyes were down to here. The bags. The bags! My face is pasty yellow, my teeth are just almost like a fluorescent greenish. You know how you leave cocaine on your mouth and it becomes numb and it starts to kill your teeth? That's what had happened to me and I couldn't put my lip down. When I talked to people they'd go, "Why are you shaking?" I'd tell them I was born with rickets.

I had a nice night, a really nice night. We all went to some hot springs and made love, woke up, and made love again. Then I said goodbye to Christopher and went to Montana with Fred and Timmy.

"They told me I never had to feel that way again."

I slept for two and a half days. In Montana I found out that I was a cocaine addict. I tried to call my cocaine connection to have him send me some drugs. I was desperate. I withdrew off the walls of my parents' house. I had no Valium. I had alcohol and we found some mushrooms. And we found some pot. When I came back from Montana I got drunk again. I wanted cocaine so bad, I was screaming. I knew I couldn't do it. I had my last use of cocaine that night.

I called Fred at four o'clock in the morning and told him I was flipping out and couldn't handle it. I was shaking so bad. I was just gone. There were ants crawling all over me. Cockroaches were invading my brain. I had a man I didn't even know sleeping upstairs in my bed. But he was a coke dealer and that was fine and I threw him out. He was drinking 180 proof grain alcohol. Oh God, I was desperate.

The next day I went to my second Cocaine Anonymous meeting. They told me I never had to feel that way again if I was willing to do one simple thing. I said, "What simple thing?" They said, "Don't drink, don't use, go to meetings and read the book." I didn't drink, I didn't use, I went to meetings, but I told them to shove their book up their a— holes. I did not do very well.

I had to go to a place called Detox to sweat the impurities out of my system. I had a hole in my nose and that got healed. My sinuses were all f—ed up. I had infections and bumps on my eyes from the LSD I used to drop in them. And I used to do some strange things with cocaine—like put it in my vagina.

I went into full-blown hallucinations, like seeing my son dead in the middle of the highway. I was flipping out, withdrawing off all these drugs. People were after me. People were dying in the middle of the street, their heads were falling off. I mean it was just horrible. I no longer wanted to feel that way, ever again. It was so painful getting sober.

I was in a treatment unit seven weeks. During that time I had strangled a person, bit someone, and had all the doors locked on me because I tore a room apart. I knew that my life could get no worse and I was willing to die. It was as simple as that. I had nowhere to go. You know—I didn't care anymore. That was my attitude. When they asked me to share or when I insisted on sharing I would say, "F— you all and die." That's where my hope was. There was no hope. Life sucks. Everything I dreamt of—making love on the beach, being with the most gorgeous man in the world, having all the coke I wanted, having all the money, having a baby: none of these things had worked. Nothing. So in my eyes there wasn't any hope.

And something happened. They loved me unconditionally. They didn't love me because my daddy had money. They didn't love me because I had big tits. They just looked at me and said, "We know how you're hurting. Keep coming back." I was going to make them hate me but the more I hated them, the more they loved me. It was as simple as that. All I had was a drug problem. And because of this drug problem, my life had become this way. I have the disease which is called chemical dependence.

In all the years of doing drugs, no one ever told me I might have a disease. Of course, I was very good with deception. I would switch entire groups of people on a weekly basis. I always knew when it was time to go, when they stopped believing my lies, like that I had lunch with the King of Arabia.

"I'm going to do the things that keep me sober."

I went through what they call "Family." I told my father that he's loved the f—ing dog he has more than any of his kids. I told my mother I never wanted to see her f—ing knitting ever again while we were talking.

I went to meetings. I got involved. I got a job. I went to work on time, fifteen minutes early. I did my work. I didn't get into the gossip. I went to my meetings. And then something hit me: I don't have a Wednesday night meeting. I'll start my own—f— it. So I started the first Cocaine Anonymous speaker meeting in this area.

One thing I wanted to do was see Christopher again. My head said no; my stomach said, you need to. And I did. I went to Christopher and I saw a different person. I saw a nice guy. And I was able to make some amends to him and not go to bed with him. So this was one of the things that gave me hope. That this slutty sleazy bitch—that's how I thought of myself—was not going to go down to that level again.

And I was willing to give my marriage one more chance because I could not go through life wondering if, now that I'm off drugs, would it have worked? So I just try. To the best of my ability. I don't medicate my child anymore. I don't spank him. I sit with him and I talk with him. I love him. I play with him. I cry with him. I don't have to tell him to get the f— out of here because I'm on coke. Or when he used to come over to give me a hug and the coke was sitting right there I couldn't because he might tip over the coke. Or when he was sitting here playing with make-believe straws saying, "This is momma's toy."

And today I'm able to look at my father and say, "I don't need you anymore. If you would like to be in my life, that's your choice."

And it is his choice. Because I'm no longer grabbing on to him like a six-year-old, begging for his attention because I feel so worthless. Because I know inside my father's not going to fix it.

I'm going to do the things that keep me sober, but if I can't, that's okay, Nanci. You know, all my life I've put these tremendous goals and expectations on myself and I've never lived up to them. I've compared my insides to other people's outsides, and because of the people I pick, the fashion ladies, I'll never measure up. Someone told me to carry my own measuring stick. Measure how I am today. The only hope that I have is, I'm getting better. That's all it is for me, knowing that I can be better today than I was yesterday.

9
Crack
Lindy's Story

The Most Addictive Drug

Cocaine is a versatile drug. You can snort it as a powder, mainline it in liquefied form, or smoke it as freebase—a more potent form of cocaine that does not dissolve in water. Until recently, the process of turning powdered cocaine into freebase was a complicated process which involved the use of volatile chemicals, such as ether, which were hard to get and dangerous to work with. Making and using freebase was limited to the more dedicated cocaine addicts.

But a few years ago an easier way was found to turn cocaine to base using only baking soda, water, and heat. After a few minutes, any kitchen chemist could easily turn powdered coke into hard rocks that were at least seventy percent pure cocaine. Those rocks have come to be called crack.

We first heard about crack in 1982. We were told it was *the* drug of choice in the black sections of Oakland. We never tried it. Three years later, crack was a phenomenon worthy of mention on the nightly news. By 1986 crack had become the nation's number one drug preoccupation and was, according to the Drug Enforcement Agency (DEA), "readily available" in major cities across America.[1] Its use spread so rapidly in these urban centers that by May, 1986, New York City had put together a force of 110 experienced narcotics officers just to fight the spread of crack.[2] In Los Angeles, more than two-thirds of cocaine arrests involve crack.[3] In some cities, crack has already become the most popular of *all* drugs.[4]

Crack is rapidly bringing cocaine addiction to a generation of young people. In an annual survey of seniors at 130 high schools, crack appeared as a "significant mode of drug taking" for the first time in 1986.[5]

For women, crack is a catastrophe. In New York City, the number of women applying for treatment at one center went from 774 in 1985 to 1349 in 1986, while the number of women seeking treatment in state-financed centers rose from twenty percent in 1980 to thirty-three percent in 1986. In both instances, much of the increase is attributed to crack.[6]

Among the black population, where more than half the families are headed by women, crack is threatening the very survival of family life. According to one doctor, crack is "such a devastating addiction that these people are willing to abandon food and water and child to take care of their crack habit."[7] In one Harlem medical center, three infants died in one six-month period in 1986, the first loss of life at the center in nearly twenty years of treating babies born to addicts.[8]

With the growing availability of crack, it seems fairly clear that its use will continue to mushroom. As increasing numbers of people, particularly youths and women, are introduced to cocaine, and as more and more snorters shift over to freebasing, crack may well become the most serious drug problem we have ever faced. As a former director of NIMH's Division of Narcotic Addiction and Drug Abuse put it, "Techniques or drugs that produce more intense and immediate effects tend to displace those that provide slower and more moderate effects."[9]

Statistics bear out this observation. According to NIDA, forty-one percent of cocaine users admitted to treatment centers during 1984 were shooting it or smoking freebase, up from twenty-five percent in 1977. In a 1985 survey of cocaine users calling the 800-COCAINE hotline, forty-eight percent were shooting or using freebase.[10] Between January and March, 1986, according to a survey of 576 hospitals across the country, fifteen percent of people admitted for cocaine-related problems had smoked crack.[11]

Crack's lure is its relatively low cost and extraordinary potency. Unlike snorted cocaine, which is absorbed through mucous membranes and arrives at the brain, greatly diluted, after five minutes, crack is absorbed directly into the lungs and hits the brain within seven seconds, producing a wallop of euphoria that is even more powerful than mainlined coke. Snorted coke produces a comparatively smooth sense of euphoria that lasts for twenty minutes to an hour. The effects of crack wear off much faster, and within minutes, crack's crash produces a craving for another puff. Developing an addiction to snorted coke might take a year or more; addiction to crack can develop in a matter of weeks.[12]

Crack addiction is tough to fight, and the helping community is responding with a variety of therapeutic techniques to help people kick the stuff, including acupuncture and the use of cocaine antidotes.[13,14] But to deal with the vicious depression and overpowering urges to go back to the drug, and to address the emotional and environmental pressures that may lead a woman to use cocaine, inpatient treatment of at least four weeks is strongly recommended.[15]

A woman who fails to stay clean despite excellent care should not be labelled a hopeless case. So powerful is crack's lure that recidivism rates are thought to be as high as ninety percent.[16] Crack addicts may need to go through a treatment program more than once.

The story that follows graphically describes one black woman's struggle with crack. And although Lindy's background was in some ways unrepresentative of many women of color, her story does introduce the woefully neglected problem of drug use among minority women.

*   *   *

Lindy's Story

Lindy is an attractive, articulate black woman whose inner strength is unmistakable. She has a determined, nononsense air about her. What impressed us most about her was her bravery in telling her story, even the painful parts, after only one year of sobriety.

I was born in Delaware, in 1953. I am an only child. I grew up in a black middle-class neighborhood and I was raised in the Pentecostal church. My upbringing was very strict and very rigid. Any time I wasn't in school, I was at church. I wasn't allowed to be like the other children. No dances, no dates, no sports, and I was only allowed friends who were in the same religion.

My father and mother had a business doing maintenance for corporate offices. As their reputation grew, their business grew and they wound up with numerous buildings throughout the city.

My mother died when I was seven years old. I was terrified by that, and sick for a while afterwards. I was raised by my grandmother, my father, and an aunt. My father, my grandmother, and myself lived together until I was fifteen when my father remarried and moved to Kentucky. I didn't get along with my stepmother, so I stayed with my grandmother. With my father out of the house, I began to change.

When I went to college I got really wild, trying to catch up on all the things that I missed and daydreamed about. I got an M.S. degree in communication and started going with a man who was ten years older than me, kind of like a father image. I ended up getting married as a way of escaping from my grandmother. I don't know why he married me. He didn't like the same things that I did, like partying. He said he loved me but we never got along. I never loved him. After about a year, we had a child.

"I told him it was medication."

I was very faithful in the beginning, to my health, to my marriage, to my husband, to my child. I put in a lot of time and energy, but felt I wasn't getting a return on my investment. I decided, "To hell with this." So I took a job with a company and I began to travel a lot. I got to where I didn't want to be at home.

I met a man in Hollywood who had lots of money and lots of cocaine. Every weekend, from Friday to Sunday, he would have crack parties. The first time he offered me a hit I didn't like it. I thought I would pass out. It made me nauseated. It gave me diarrhea and totally took away my appetite. So for a time I just sat and watched other people do it. After the nauseous feeling left me I tried it again. Once I got to like it, it was like nothing else had ever made me that euphoric. Nothing could give me that feeling, I mean absolutely nothing.

I began to do it pretty consistently right from the start. My friend would give me coke to take home and I learned how to make crack. I'd mix the ingredients in a test tube, boil it and swirl it, and there it was. Crack. Rock hard. I'd take a razor blade and cut it into the small parts, and put it on my freebase pipe, and put a torch to it made of a cotton ball dipped in alcohol. As the crack melts, I'm inhaling as much smoke as I can, holding it in.

I stayed in Hollywood for six or seven months, then I'd go back to my husband and daughter for awhile. I brought my habit home with me. I was draining our bank account right down, one hundred dollars every couple of days, deceiving myself by buying a little at a time. I liquidated insurance policies, you know, like thousands of dollars. My husband was so dumb straight he didn't know anything about me and crack. I'd go into the bathroom, take my vial and paraphernalia, and cook it right there. I'd set my pipe up in a drawer and every once in a while duck into the room and take a hit and then that hit would—I'd feel so wonderful. I don't think I acted any differently. Maybe a little hyper, but that's the way I am anyway.

I cooked it up in front of my husband once. I told him it was the medication that had been prescribed by the doctor. He believed me, until he talked to a friend who told him, "Man your wife is doing drugs—she's doing crack." And he came back and confronted me. I didn't try to hide it. I gave him all kinds of reasons why I did it. But he was probably very upset about the amount of money that I had gone through, thousands and thousands of dollars. I stopped taking the money out of the account, and I started spending even more of the year on the West Coast.

"I was chasing an illusion that I never caught."

At that point I didn't consider myself addicted. I could go two or three days, or even two or three weeks, without smoking crack. But once I became addicted, doing it every day, things got really bad and I lost everything. I had no pride, no dignity left. I would go to the worst area, to crack houses where people were sitting on the doorway with guns. I've been in so many horrible situations I can't even tell them all. At times I needed cocaine so badly I'd wind up in crack houses with two guys with machine guns sitting at the door and me propped in the corner hitting a pipe, you know, and not fazed by the police running up and down the street outside or the chance of them busting in any moment.

I was doing things that were totally unlike me, morally and every other way. I had lost control of my life. I'd leave my house, supposedly going to a store which was thirty minutes away, and I'd end up being gone for days. And for that whole time I'd be out freebasing. In my last episode I had told the people I was living with that I was going to the store and I didn't come back for six days. When they found me I was in a semicomatose state and I hadn't eaten or drunk anything since I had left.

At a certain point my rich Hollywood connection got busted with about $180,000 worth of cocaine, so I had to start associating with people in the ghetto, in the crack houses. But once I opened my mouth, those people knew I was different. That created a lot of hostility.

And, you know, I was a prime candidate for getting involved with men. They found me attractive and sophisticated, unlike most of the women that were there. There were times that I felt attracted to some of them and wanted to be intimate and sometimes I didn't. Whenever I found the situation hostile, I had sense enough to leave. But I only left to find it someplace else. I seemed to only want to be involved with men who either had a lot of money or had access to a lot of drugs.

My life just became totally unmanageable. I started by freebasing on weekends, then went to doing it after work. I ended up doing it from the moment I got off work to the next morning. I could never take just one hit 'cause one hit would make me want another, and another, and another. I was chasing that original hit, constantly pumping it into my system. I was chasing an illusion that I never caught.

"I didn't know I was addicted."

I was strung out every morning. I once tried smoking a joint to calm me down, but it sent me into a seizure and I had to go to the hospital. Well, actually, I went to the hospital lots of times. Once I had been freebasing for maybe two days and I was in this guy's heart-shaped pool, smoking a joint. I began to feel funny. I passed out. He took me to the hospital. My pulse was so low they couldn't find it for a while. I stayed in for two days.

There are a lot of things I just can't go into, because they're just too horrible to try to recall. I was involved in a love triangle and . . . well, the bottom line is that the the guy tricked me into coming to his home by telling me he was sick and needed my help. When I went to his house, he opened the door, snatched me, and choked me till I was unconscious. When I came to he had a gun to my head, demanding the answers to a lot of questions I couldn't answer. He was crying and disoriented. He cocked the trigger. I don't know why he didn't pull it. I guess I'm living and breathing and alive today only because God was merciful. I have no other explanations for it at all.

When I compared the way I was raised and the person I was before being involved with the drugs with what I had become, it was like I didn't recognize myself anymore. Once I was at a party, the only woman in a room with fifteen men. Everybody in that room had a freebase pipe in their hand, and then the police came crashing through the door, guns drawn. I might have been different from everyone in the room, but I went to jail just the same.

I was so ashamed. I sat there for three days. I couldn't call anyone, I couldn't explain why I was there. I didn't want my respected, professional, sophisticated friends to know where I was. At that time I had lost a good amount of weight. Now I'm 130 pounds. I was 104 pounds then. I think I hadn't bathed for a week. I was awful. I was just awful. I can't tell you how badly I felt. Badly! Badly doesn't even come close to the humiliation I felt. I felt like I didn't deserve to live. I couldn't understand what was making me live like this. I still didn't know I was addicted.

And as I sat there in jail a police officer who was a friend of mine was on duty that very night. And I saw her and I wanted to hide but I was in a cage, right in everybody's view. She saw me and she came to me and said, "What are you doing here? What's wrong? Look at you." She talked to me and I told her, "I can't tell anyone where I am." She convinced me to call for help. I couldn't tell my family on the East Coast. I called my roommate. She mortgaged some property to put up for my bail to get me out of jail. And she nurtured me back to health.

"I took the kid with me."

So for a while I got off crack, but I went right back. I didn't understand what was happening to me. I didn't understand why I had this powerlessness, this drive, this compulsion that made me do everything I was always against. Cocaine drives you—the compulsion to use is greater than any other drug because no other drug makes you feel that happy. Anything can be wrong, you know. When my father died, I took the biggest pipe and I freebased and it seemed all right. I mean it makes everything all right.

Once I was babysitting a five-year-old child for a friend. I had to go to the store so I took the child with me, just because I wanted to assure myself—this is how bad my habit had gone— that I *would* go to the store and come right back home. I didn't. I took the child. I had the money. I said I'll just go get me just a small chip, a quarter rock.

I did the quarter and it got me started. A habit can never do a little bit. You know the little bit only gets you started. I had no more money. I had to go around begging, from friend to friend, from crack house to crack house. I never bothered going back home. Of course, the kid's parents called the police. I was on the news. I was freebasing for days, driving around with the kid hidden in my car, police all around me. I took care of the kid, kept him fed and all. I'd take him to the crack houses with me and sit him in a corner near some guy with a machine gun or something.

After four days of this, of doing crack and not sleeping, I called a friend and asked if I could come over to her house. By this time the whole world is looking for me. I told her, "Look, don't tell anyone anything and when I get there, I'll turn you on." She told me she wouldn't tell anyone. Meanwhile, she calls a friend who comes in when I'm getting high. This friend calls the kid's mother, who comes over and gets her child. Once they got the child back and realized it was unharmed, the police dropped any charges. They realized I hadn't meant any harm. I was just out of it.

"I didn't want to wake up to the reality of what I had done."

I mean, that was only the 100th or 150th thing that I had done that was totally disastrous. But when you're strung out or hung up on drugs you don't talk rationally. You just continue to use. I knew I had done an awful thing in taking the kid with me in the first place, and in order to stop that depression I continued to get high. I realized how much trouble I was in. So it was like—run, hide, and just stay high. And that's what I did.

Eventually I reached a point where I realized this could not go on. Once, after I had been on a six-day binge, I knew I was dying. I kept fading out of it. I hadn't eaten—I was down to like ninety some pounds from 130. It was like I was either going to freebase myself to death or somebody was going to help. I had done so much harm to so many people. I was so depressed. I just didn't want to wake up to the reality of what I had done. I had gone from being a very moral, ultrasophisticated, very well respected, successful black lady to smack dead in the middle of a ghetto, looking like the worst bum that you could ever imagine. Then a friend, this guy who was really in love with me, found me and took me to a hospital. And from the hospital I went to a rehab center.

I didn't want to be at the Center. I had gained some weight and had gotten stabilized by the time I was released from the hospital and I was told I'd live provided I didn't use. I was in the Center for eight days when I got an overpowering urge to have another hit. I had to have it. So I called a dealer and made arrangements for him to pick me up on my four-hour pass. I was going to smoke some crack and go right back to the Center and everything would be fine. I went out, I used, and I couldn't stop. I didn't go back to the Center. And this time it finally hit me. Everything over the past five years—the near brushes with death, the number of people's lives I had made total catastrophes of, the jail scenes, and my child. She came to visit me lots of times and I was totally a wreck. I mean I used to disappear for three, four, or five days at a time. She wouldn't see me, she wouldn't hear from me.

You know, I told my daughter I had a habit and that I needed help. And I sat and talked to her and we both cried for hours. And she said "Mother, I'll do anything I can to help you." She said "I want you to get some help." I had gotten down to three or four cracks, three or four hits left, and I hit them. Then I cracked the pipe and threw it away. I threw it away and called the hospital and asked them, begged them, to let me come back in. This time I went in on my own. This time I really wanted help and to be free from the habit. I did.

"And when that physical urge to use crack comes back . . ."

When I had gone in the first time, I was very resentful. And after my relapse I lied to them. I told them I hadn't used, and made up some wild story about why I had left the hospital. But I ended up accepting the program and realizing in order for me to achieve what I wanted, which was sobriety, I was going to have to conform to the things that the program had proven very viable. After a while I adjusted. I was in there for two months. It was an extended time, but I needed that time.

I had incredible urges at first, my whole body craved another hit. There were times when the craving was so bad I could just sit in the corner and stay there. Then I'd call my sponsor or go to an AA meeting or read my Bible. Go to church. But reach out. And when things get rough, when things get really bad—things that I would have avoided or used as an excuse to go out and get high over—now I take another avenue of escape. You know—I pray. I go to church. I go to AA meetings. I stand up and I talk to crowds and I tell them how I'm feeling and that's how I got my year.

I take sobriety a day at a time, or sometimes it has to be an hour at a time. A week before Thanksgiving I lost a stepsister. There would have been a time I'd have used that as an excuse to smoke crack to the point of death. Now I pray. And I go to church and I reach out and I ask for help. I get on my knees. And when that physical urge to use crack comes back, then I use the tools I learned at the center, and they work. If you'll follow the Twelve Steps it works, it works.

"I stay in touch with people who are positive influences."

I can never say I will be sober for the rest of my life. I can say I want to be sober for the rest of my life on a daily basis, and that assures my sobriety. Today I'm sober and I'm happy. This was the first Christmas and New Year I've been sober for five or six years. And it's really incredible. My daughter was here for the Christmas holiday and we had an incredible time. I thank God that I wasn't on drugs and I feel good about it. My minister called me yesterday morning and I stay in touch with people who are positive influences in my life.

A lot of people I went through the program with are doing drugs again. You really have to want to be sober. And in some ways fighting drugs is easier now. The government is taking drugs more seriously. People are getting more educated about them. Sometimes an urge to do drugs would come over me and maybe at the same time an announcement is coming on TV where somebody is saying, "I had a house and I had children and I had a good job," and he says, "I lost it all because I used cocaine." There is a constant reminder on television, on radio, in magazines, which is wonderful now.

The hardest part of getting clean was having to confess a lot of things I did and lies I told, and having to tell that to my daughter. Having to tell them to people who were close to me. And also winning the confidence of the people back, convincing them that I really wanted to be sober and having to deal with their lack of trust. Because, what can I expect? I used to say, "I'm going to the store," and I'd be gone for five or six days. When I first became sober, if I walked out of the house to the store there would be doubt and all this mistrust. And if I didn't come back at a certain time, they'd ask, "Did you go out and use?" That's very hard.

"My goal is to be a responsible person again."

I'm starting to save money again. Before, whenever I had a little money, I'd take it to buy coke. I've been offered crack. I can say, "No, I don't do drugs." And that's what makes me happy. To know that I really am sincere about it. Because I remember a time when I couldn't have said no. I know I can never take the first hit, because the first one would lead ultimately to my death. I'd be so disappointed with myself for relapsing that the amount I would need to consume to bury the depression probably would kill me. So I don't even want the first hit. You know, at the center they told us that when the urge comes over you, think of all the bad things that happened, and that takes the desire away. I know that the low is so so so so low.

I'm happy about my job, my life is coming together. A lot of the things I couldn't do because of my addiction I'm doing now. I've spent more time with my daughter probably in the last year than in the previous five years. Because I'm here. You know. All the time before was spent in the crack house or somewhere getting high, and that's a lot of time. The time that's involved in freebasing is a lot of time because you cook it and then you smoke it and then you have to go get some more. Doing crack, you're a slave to a room and to a pipe and you don't go anywhere. You don't leave it because you're afraid someone is going to take your part of it. It's incredible what a slave you are to the drug. You're strapped. Absolutely strapped.

My goal is to be a responsible person again. To prove that and to know and to see the confidence that people gain in me along the way. People see that I've changed. They know that I'm different. And that's wonderful.

But the best thing was that I got honest. You have to get honest. Honesty is just ultimately important. You can't do anything without honesty. You must get totally honest. I divulged things I don't even want God to know, and that's pretty hard to do. It was very humbling to realize I can't do it alone, that I needed help and had to reach out and get it.

10

Crystal Sissy's Story

Life on a Rollercoaster

Crystal, the most potent form of speed, first appeared in the early sixties during the opening stages of the American amphetamine epidemic.[1] Injectable ampules of methamphetamine had just been outlawed and thousands of speed addicts were left without a legal supply of their drug. Crystal quickly filled the gap.

Crystal was—and is—surprisingly easy to make. All the ingredients can be purchased legally from chemical supply houses and it doesn't take a genius to cook it up. By the late sixties, five to ten labs on the West Coast were turning out twenty-five to one hundred pounds of crystal a week.[2]

While no one can say with certainty how much crystal is being manufactured today, in one Southwest city alone enough chemical precursors are sold to make eleven thousand pounds of crystal a year.[3] The 479 methamphetamine labs seized by the law enforcement agencies in 1986 probably represent only a small fraction of the labs that continue to operate.[4] Crystal makers are more than willing to take high risks for enormous profits: a one-thousand-dollar investment can yield forty thousand dollars' return.[5]

Women were part of crystal's spread from the beginning, both as users *and* movers. By 1969, there were documented reports of one nine-year-old girl running a bathtub lab in her home and another fifteen-year-old girl mixing up batches with twenty dollars' worth of equipment.[6,7]

Whether it's snorted or dissolved in water and shot intravenously, crystal produces behavior which more nearly fits the popular idea of "dope fiend" than even heroin: bizarre actions, compulsiveness, emaciation and fearfulness.[8] And though "speed freaks" are usually pictured as men, more than a third of the crystal abusers who wind up in emergency rooms are female, as are more than a quarter who wind up in the medical examiner's morgue.[9]

Crystal is not generally considered an addictive drug, but its effects are initially so deeply gratifying, it can hook a woman as quickly and as thoroughly as heroin can.[10] In fact, the likelihood that a user will eventually progress from controlled to compulsive use is thought to be much higher with crystal than with any other substance.[11] In some cities, the number of intravenous speed users may equal the number of heroin users.[12]

We can look at the cycle of crystal addiction as a series of four clearly marked stages.

First, a woman trying crystal usually starts out by snorting it for an exciting mood lift. She feels an instant improvement in self-image[13]. Even if she's normally reticent and shy, she'll lose her inhibitions and appear spontaneous, sociable, and witty, becoming the party person she always wanted to be.[14] Any crash she experiences at this stage is only mildly unpleasant.

After awhile she grows dependent on this chemical lift and finds that tooting it no longer takes her where she wants to go. To get that magic rush in the briefest time, she has to progress to crystal's second stage: mainlining.[15]

Shooting crystal is typically done in runs: continuous use every few hours for several days, followed by a period of sleep.[16] Shooting crystal gives a woman an intensely hedonistic rush. She feels as if her entire being has experienced a kind of orgasm. Everything she does, everything that happens to her, has an immediacy, an importance, and an excitement to it.

The third stage of crystal use marks the beginning of rapid decline, the familiar "going down from here" that several users told us about. By now, tolerance to both the psychological and physical effects of crystal force a woman to increase her dose as the run progresses. The big ecstasy is always one more syringe-full away. Often she will "overamp," taking more crystal than ever in a desperate attempt to reach that elusive original high. By the fifth day of a run, however, no amount of crystal can take the shooter where she wants to go.[17]

By the fourth stage her mental and physical condition have deteriorated, and the crash that follows each run now becomes unbearable. She suffers from immobilizing depression and lethargy and will typically turn to tranquilizers or barbiturates to sleep through the worst of it.

Soon after awakening, the woman is ready to shoot again. Each subsequent run may fail to get her as high as her first, but each will surely leave her even lower than the last. The flash of euphoria and exhiliration she experiences at the beginning of each run can only temporarily hide the devastation that crystal is wreaking on her mind and body. Weight loss leads to emaciation and malnutrition. Excitement gives way to abdominal cramping and chest pains. Her sociability turns to lonely hours spent grinding her teeth while she picks at the "bugs" crawling under her skin. Continued high IV doses lead to liver disease, strokes, injury to her arteries and veins, and brain damage.[18]

Even more alarming is the way in which speed causes a woman's personality to deteriorate. Once the rush is over, she goes through rapid changes of mood; she feels paranoid, hallucinates, hears voices, imagines she is being watched by people she cannot see, and comes to believe that others—neighbors, strangers, the CIA—can read her mind. Her thinking becomes confused and disorganized. Her reactions often become so aggressive and violent that stable, supportive relationships become impossible. She feels estranged and alienated from everyone.

Speed's downward plunge leads finally to temporary psychosis, characterized by repetition of nonsensical phrases, screaming, and suicidal ideas. No matter how psychologically sound a speed user is at the beginning of her drug use, given enough crystal over enough time, she will become psychotic.[19]

A woman kicking her habit needs lots of support and guidance to rebuild her physical health and return to psychological normalcy. She needs to be welcomed back to ordinary society as a participating member of a peer support group. Perhaps more than with any other drug, the former crystal user, accustomed to sleepless nights, needs access to support on a twenty-four-hour-a-day basis.[20] As horrible and dehumanizing as the speed experience is, there is little doubt that most addicts, if not all, can bounce back from even the most

profound intellectual disorganization and psychosis after six months
or a year of sobriety.[21]

In the strictest sense, the slogan of the sixties—Speed Kills—
was more frightening than accurate. Even after sizable overdoses,
crystal is rarely fatal. But it is lethal in other ways. In 1969 we moved
to the Haight-Ashbury in San Francisco, hoping to catch the tail
end of the love generation. What we saw resembled a city under
siege. Shop windows were boarded up, streets were deserted at night
and, instead of smiles and songs, we found snarls and fear. The
psychedelic movement had been laid waste by speed, and we
understood how speed killed.

We didn't meet up with speed again until the late seventies. A
friend of ours, we learned, had been tooting it occasionally, and
then shooting it frequently. We noticed remarkable changes in her.
We saw her joy of life vanish, and watched her face and eyes take
on a desperate, frightened, hungry look. She became increasingly
fearful of everyone and told us when she lay quietly in bed she could
hear people in nearby houses talking about her. She lost her job, her
roommates, and her home. Her lover tried to get her medical help
but she had no insurance, so she was bundled off to a county mental
ward which offered her only short-term care for her symptoms.
After detoxing, she was released, and went back to speed and her
terrible torments. One day we learned she had ended her suffering
by cutting her wrists.

The story that follows is no less harrowing, but has a happier
ending.

*   *   *

Sissy's Story

*When we met Sissy, she was eighteen years old and had
been clean and sober about one year. She was a curious
mixture of adolescent enthusiasm and mature restraint,
and she looked the picture of health. She was eager to
tell us her story, she said, because she was just doing her
Fourth Step in AA, which states, "We made a searching
and fearless moral inventory of ourselves."*

I was born on October 3, 1969. My dad is a drug counselor in the
Air Force and my mom's a school nurse. My mom and dad didn't
drink or take drugs, but my mom is bulimic. My dad's father was
an alcoholic, and my mom's dad died of an overdose of Valium.

Because my dad was in the Air Force, we moved around from
place to place to place when I was a child and I had a real hard time
making friends. I was really fat as a kid and I developed a complex
about it. My mother was always saying, "Oh Sissy, you shouldn't
be eating that food." Kids were so mean, always making fun of fat
people. I used to go home crying all the time.

I never fit in with other girls. I had a violent attitude and I did
things that guys do, like spit and beat up other kids. I got really
good in sports, to please my dad, who used to be a football player.

"I'd get stoned before I went to school in time for lunch."

I started drinking when I was in the sixth grade. I'd come home
from school and I would get into my parents' liquor cabinet, which
they kept for company, and drink and act silly by myself. One night
two friends dared me to drink a shot of everything in the liquor
cabinet. There must have been fifty bottles of stuff and I got really
drunk. I jumped to the bottom of the pool and just sat there until I
passed out. I guess my friends pulled me out, but I don't remember.

From the time I was eleven I started hanging out with kids who
were much older than me, like eighteen and nineteen. I told them I

was sixteen and they believed me. We used to buy beer and get drunk. One day they asked me, "Have you ever tried pot?" I said, "Sure, but I don't like it." They offered me a joint and said, "Try this." I was really scared, but I started smoking so I could fit in with them.

I got into some real uncomfortable situations with older guys. Once I was almost raped. This guy took me on a walk and started touching me. I told him to stop and he said, "Come on, you know you want it." I started screaming and he grabbed me and pulled me to the ground. He just wouldn't stop touching. I kicked him as hard as I could and ran away. I was really terrified, but I couldn't tell anyone about it.

I got passing grades in school, but I was always getting into trouble for talking back to my teachers. If one of them said, "I told you you need to pay attention in my class," I'd say, "I can do anything I damn well please in this class." I really had a big mouth. I didn't care how old or big or important someone was, I'd mouth off at them if I felt like it. All my friends' parents banned me from seeing their kids because I had a reputation as a smart ass. Like if some girl was having a birthday party, you could bet I was not allowed on her guest list.

By the seventh grade a typical day for me would be to have some wine and get stoned before I went to school in time for lunch. Then I'd smoke some more down by the bushes where some of the kids hung out, and sort of sleep the day away. My parents were kind of suspicious, but if they ever said anything I'd just yell at them, "Goddamn it, you people don't trust me!"

"The kids in the twelfth grade knew where to get the better stuff."

Me and my dad used to get into really violent fights. If they complained about something that I had done at school—like telling a teacher to go f— herself—I'd tell my dad that if he hadn't moved around so much, I would have had some friends and if my mother hadn't taught me such bad eating habits I wouldn't be so goddamned fat. Then my dad would say, "Don't use that foul language with me," and I'd go, "I'll say whatever I f—ing well want to." Then he would smack me and I'd smack him back. Then my mom would get in my face and try to break in, so I'd smack her, and he'd smack me for hitting her. I think that happened three or four times a week. I used to go to school with bruises on me.

My father never touched my brother, who was a really good kid, kind of what they call the lost child in psychology. When my parents and I fought, he'd just disappear into his room and work on his computer. I tried to get him to take drugs, because I thought if he did, I'd be able to get away with a lot more stuff. Some friends and I once forced a bong in his mouth, but he wouldn't smoke it. So I slapped him around. I have to admit he really saved my butt a lot. I'd be so wasted after my parties that he'd be the one to clean everything up so my parents and I wouldn't fight.

I got introduced to crystal in the seventh grade, from the same friends who dared me to drink all the alcohol. They asked if I wanted to try it and I said sure. I got a hold of twenty-five dollars and we waited in a parking lot for our connection to show. He drove up on a motorcycle, took my money and threw a little package wrapped in newspaper into the car. It was a capsule filled with crystal. I snorted it like my friends showed me to do and I got kind of wired. But I didn't think it was that good. I wanted to try better stuff.

I started hanging around with kids in the eleventh and twelfth grades who knew where to get better stuff. I'd go to their parties and act really cool, popping into the bathroom to do a few lines. I felt really confident on speed. I loved being able to go up to all these people I had always felt insecure with and just talk to them. I got a lot of attention and I couldn't shut up. At school I'd tell the other kids what I did the night before, how much I partied, and they'd just say, "Wow." I felt like I was the greatest thing on earth, like I was really loved.

From the outside, speed made me look good. I lost twenty-five pounds. I started cleaning my room, then I started cleaning the whole house. My mom said, "God, I don't know what's happened to you but I like you so much better."

"I was sleeping with guys for the stuff."

By the eighth grade I was smoking pot and drinking every day, and doing crystal whenever I could get it. I'd ask someone at school, "Do you have any crystal?" Then we'd go in the bathroom and do it. I was stealing money from my parents constantly, taking twenty bucks at a time for drugs.

It was at this time I first had sex with a guy. All my girlfriends were telling me how they always had sex. None of them really did, but I believed them. One night I decided I was going to get really drunk at a party and do it. I started talking to this one guy and we went into an empty bedroom and did it right there. Afterwards, he just dumped me. He left. I was really upset, because that wasn't the way it was supposed to be. So I went back to the party and drank about a quart of vodka and started rapping with another guy. We left the party and went to the restroom of a gas station and had sex there. Then he dumped me, too. I got a reputation at school for being a slut, and all my friends dropped me.

I was so angry, and lonely. I didn't understand why life was so tough. I didn't have anyone I could turn to. When I wasn't partying, I'd sit alone in my room talking to my dog. I used to fall asleep at night, crying, feeling like there was this big hole in my heart. It hurt so bad.

When I got out of eighth grade my parents decided I needed to see a psychologist because I was having problems. They were fine, I was sick. The psychologist decided my father was a child abuser and needed help. That was a shock. I had never thought of that before. I didn't like seeing the psychologist. My mother started going with me, and she didn't like him either. We started bullsh—ting him together. My mother would tell me, "Don't tell him about the fight we had. Just say everything's all right." After a little while, we stopped going to him.

By the end of ninth grade I was doing lots of crystal. I was sleeping with guys for the stuff and I was doing it seven days a week. I'd get money for it any way I could think of, I don't even remember how. Every morning I'd wake up and think, "How am I going to get crystal today?" I told two of my boyfriends I needed money for abortions. I hocked some of my parents' things. I stole from friends. I slept with guys who were using, too. That was the easiest way to get it. I always went for the guys with girlfriends, because I hated girls. I used to rub it in their faces—"I slept with your boyfriend."

I was always going through these powerful mood swings every eight days that my parents didn't understand. I was crashing was what was happening. I looked disgusting. My skin was a gross yellow. I'd pick at my skin because I thought I had bugs underneath. When my nose bled from too much snorting, I told my mother I had a cold. When my face broke out in blotches, I told her it was too much sun.

"I'd go to the park and buy needles from the bums."

I got really paranoid, too. I was always sure there were people outside my window. I stopped walking around my house in my underwear because I was sure people were watching me. I used to think that people had put video cameras in my room, and whenever I hid my stash I was sure they saw where I hid it. I got to where I just kept my stash on me.

In the tenth grade I joined a punk circle. I dyed my hair outrageous colors, had my nose pierced. All I had to do to have friends was be mean and take lots of drugs. I met a girl who told me she shot crystal. "It's so cool because you get ten times more wired," she said. Did I want to do it? Of course I did.

I never experienced anything like it before. I was wired for three days. I had to wear long-sleeve shirts because of a bruise on my arm. I thought, "This is great: It's cheaper, it's stronger, it's easier, it doesn't burn my nose." And I felt tougher. My goal was now to be the biggest drug addict that ever lived and the biggest dealer. I just started going downhill.

I started doing about a gram and a half a day. I just couldn't stop. I had lumps in my arm. I thought it was going to fall off. I'd go to the park and buy needles from the bums for two dollars each. They were used, but I figured they were only used once so there was no problem. I didn't know you could get AIDS from them. I just didn't think I'd get sick. And I didn't care if I lived or died anyway.

One night a bunch of us were sitting in an abandoned shack, a really disgusting place, shooting up. I took too much and suddenly I couldn't breathe; my chest felt like it was caving in. "I want to go to a doctor," I told them. And everybody said, "No, no, we can't get busted." So I sat there all night. I thought I was dying.

I developed twitches from speed. I felt dirty. I would scrub and scrub in the shower, but I never felt clean enough. So I just stopped taking showers. My hair became so matted, I told my mother it was part of the style. I used to pull my hair out, too.

In school I would just sit there and vege out, thinking how stupid everyone else was. I didn't talk to anyone. At home I'd barely say a word to my parents. My brother knew I was doing drugs and he threatened to tell on me, so I'd knock him around the house. All I wanted to do was be bad.

"He slapped me around and raped me."

I was always being busted for being out after curfew. One night I was hanging around the park, really drunk and high, and these men came over to me and said they wanted to see some ID. I said, "F— you, show me *your* ID." They pulled out their badges and I heard their walkie talkies. They took me down to Juvenile Hall. They said I looked like a hooker, I told them they looked like faggots. "You're real tough, aren't you," one of them said. "You bet your a— I am," I answered. "I think you've had a terrible life," he said. "You don't know the half of it," I told him. They told me to lift up my shirtsleeves. I did and they saw the tracks. They asked me what that was from. "Crystal," I told them. They put me in the holding tank till next day when my parents came to pick me up. They never told my parents about my tracks. I told my mother I was just picked up for loitering, and she believed me.

I stopped using crystal for about a month and just kept myself fried on LSD. Then I went back to crystal again. I had this dealer who ripped me off, so I broke into his house with a couple of friends and we stole everything we could lay our hands on. I was sitting at school by myself the next day and he came over to me at school and started screaming at me. "Why are you wearing long sleeves in the summer?" "Because I'm cold," I said. "Why don't you tell everybody how you shoot up? Why don't you tell everybody what a drug fiend you are?" He kept yelling at me all over the school. I got put on restriction by my parents.

A couple of nights later, I'm sitting alone in my room, when there's a knock on my window. It's the ex-boyfriend of a girlfriend of mine. He said, "I'm on my way to a party, let me come in for awhile." "I'm not feeling too well," I told him. "Look," he said, "I've got some lines I want to do before I go to the party." So I let him in and we do some lines and he said, "Let's have sex." I said, "Are you crazy, my parents are home." But he wasn't taking no for an answer. I got really scared. I couldn't scream. I couldn't move or do anything. It's like when an earthquake happens. All I could think was, God, please get me through this. He slapped me around and raped me. He stayed five hours.

Three nights later he came back. I locked my window and didn't open it. I just couldn't walk down the hall and tell my parents, so I called a friend and told her about it. My friend tells her mother, who calls my parents. My mom called the cops. I go to the hospital and all these cops are asking me questions about the rape, telling me I could press charges if I wanted to but it would be my word against his.

"I have to remember that not all men are out to hurt me."

The next day I went to the school psychologist. I had been seeing her for years, but I never told her what was really going on. I would make up stuff that was completely opposite from my real life. That day she said, "Sissy, your mother told me you're on drugs." I just looked at her and said, "Yes, it's true." The next day my parents put me into a treatment hospital. I went through all the motions, like going to meetings and saying, "My name is Sissy and I'm an addict," not because I believed it, but because I knew that's what they wanted to hear. I stayed there a couple of weeks, but as soon as I got out I started seeing one of my ex-boyfriends and I began dealing and using again and getting really strung out.

So I went to another hospital, in an adolescent program that took six weeks. As soon as I went in, I lost all my rights. They wouldn't let me sleep when I wanted to, they wouldn't give me aspirin for my headache.

We had family group, too. I talked about the way my dad treats me, and how I thought there was something wrong with my mom and dad's relationship, because she confides in me but not in him. My dad had to deal with these things. I've seen him cry about three times since I got clean. I never saw him cry before.

My parents had to learn to not concentrate on me, because I'm not the problem. It's been a family disease, not a moral deficiency.

We all learned about denial and about dealing with our feelings. No one ever taught my mom and dad about feelings, about letting the walls down. I learned how to be me, that it was okay to feel, and to tell my feelings.

I started getting principles back, and I started loving people again, just the way they were. The program had me make up a list of how I was going to keep myself busy during the day instead of going home and sleeping and eating. They told me to write a phone list of people I could call if I needed help.

My father goes to counseling now and he's doing the best he can. I've developed really close relationships with about four or five other people from high school who are recovering. We go to meetings together, and talk about spirituality and things.

Right now I'm in a relationship with a man. I have to remember sometimes that not all men are out to hurt me, and I have to cop to my resentments against men, like my father, and all the boyfriends who dumped me. I'm still afraid that men will only like me if I have sex with them, or they're not going to like me because I'm overweight. My boyfriend keeps telling me he likes me just the way I am, but I have trouble hearing it sometimes.

I go to college and most of the people there are into heavy partying. All they talk about is drinking and getting stoned and how they couldn't make it through school without getting wired. So I have to be real careful. When I first got clean I would tell people I was a drug addict. I used to think I'd get some sympathy. I don't tell people anymore. I just try to be me. It's hard sometimes to deal with normal people. I expect them to be more feeling.

I'm really grateful that I got sober. I could never comprehend that life could be like this. I always thought I was a really hard person, and I'm not at all. I have about twenty recovering friends I can call any time of the night. And I have a sponsor.

11

Heroin
Kit's Story

In Its Wake: AIDS, Prostitution, and Stigma

Although the heroin scare of the midseventies seems far behind us, and the snowballing of cocaine use has pushed all other drugs off the front page, the surprising fact is that we are once again in the midst of a heroin epidemic.[1] Americans consumed almost six metric tons of heroin in 1984, an increase of fifty-five percent over 1981.[2] At parties all across America, heroin is riding the wave of cocaine chic. It is just one more white powder to be snorted, smoked, and shot.

Of the estimated five hundred thousand heroin addicts in this country, more than one hundred thousand are women.[3,4] An additional one million may be "chippers," women who use heroin intermittently but are not addicted, yet.[5] Heroin addiction now seems to be growing at a faster rate among women than men.[6]

Our own experience with heroin was definitely chipping. In the early seventies an artist friend offered to get us a ten-dollar bag. Our curiosity made us say yes. We snorted a couple of lines and got sick. Over the next few months, we bought a few more bags, always got sick, and always hated it. Many women are not so lucky.

Heroin abuse affects women in two tragic ways. First, heroin, often in combination with alcohol, is the number one cause of drug-related deaths among women in America. In 1984, heroin claimed an estimated three thousand lives, a rise of almost thirty percent over 1983.[7] Women comprised twenty-five percent of those deaths.

Second, more than any other drug, heroin brings to the woman addict a lifestyle of crime and degradation. In one study, seventy percent of the women in a New York City jail on a given day were heroin users. Only forty-two percent of the men were. In another study of sixty-six women addicts released from prison, after four years, two-thirds had been rearrested for drugs and stealing, seven had died from overdoses, and one had committed suicide.[8] In the course of their lives, nearly half of all female heroin addicts become full-time prostitutes, with most using it as their primary means of support at some point.[9]

Compounding this tragedy, nearly all female addicts are of childbearing age, between fifteen and thirty-five years old. And the birthrate among addicts is actually higher than it is in the general population. In 1973, the average family size for an addicted woman was 2.7 children, compared to two children for a nonaddicted woman. In that year an estimated 234,000 children had heroin-addicted mothers.[10] Today, eight out of one thousand children born in New York City are drug addicted, five times the number of twenty years ago.[11]

Heroin addiction hits black and Hispanic women especially hard. Two-thirds of the women who died from heroin in 1984 were nonwhite.[12] Ten years ago, blacks and Hispanics made up only sixteen percent of the general population but comprised seventy-five percent of the addict population.[13]

But here again, the figures are in flux. Heroin's entrenchment in the inner city ghettos may one day be seen as mere detour. In the early years of this century, women opiate addicts outnumbered men two to one.[14] The typical opiate addict was a middle-aged, middle-class Southern white woman who got her fix from any number of perfectly legal sources: doctor, drugstore or mail-order catalog. When the Harrison Act of 1914 made opium products illegal, majority Americans dropped their syringes. Now heroin is coming back home to mainstream America. From 1979 to 1985 nearly fifty percent of heroin initiates were white, and at present more white heroin initiates are entering treatment centers than blacks or Hispanics.[15,16]

And now a wild card has been added to the present epidemic that threatens to make it the most lethal and socially significant outbreak of all times: AIDS. Intravenous drug use is the number one route of AIDS transmission among women. More than half of all women with AIDS contracted it from sharing needles.[17] And according to the Centers for Disease Control, minority women are especially at risk. A Hispanic woman is eleven times more likely than a white woman to get AIDS; a black woman is at thirteen times the risk. And, because so many female addicts are prostitutes, some researchers fear that AIDS may be rapidly spreading from them into the so-called general population.[18] In a 1987 study researchers at the Centers for Disease Control found that more than eleven percent of prostitutes tested positive for the AIDS virus. In some urban areas, as many as fifty-seven percent were infected.[19]

Because politicians and moralists are reluctant to seem soft on the issues of crime and moral degradation that surround heroin addiction, rational decisions affecting heroin use and abuse have been rendered well-nigh impossible. In 1985, for instance, the U.S. House of Representatives rejected a measure that would have permitted physicians to prescribe heroin to ease the pain of terminally-ill cancer patients. Opponents of the bill argued that legal heroin might be diverted to illegal use. The maximum quantity of heroin involved was fifteen pounds a year. In that same year Mexico alone produced thirty-seven thousand pounds.[20]

A woman trying to kick heroin needs treatment, but even in treatment it's often an uphill struggle. If she has been involved in prostitution, she faces stigmatization by other clients. If she is responsible for the welfare of her children, as a large majority of drug-dependent women are, she must somehow balance those responsibilities with the tough jobs of getting clean and learning new skills.[21] Even in those enlightened communities which offer residential programs that house mother and children together, the wait for an available slot can be excruciatingly long.[22]

Heroin addiction among women is an enormously complicated problem. And it's emotionally confusing, too. The female heroin user comes smack up against our idealized vision of the perfect woman. The woman strung out on heroin seems to lack will power, probity and virtue. But seeing heroin addicts as hopelessly lost does nothing to encourage a wise solution. The story that follows may help to humanize our view of heroin-addicted women.

Finally, Kit's story introduces another issue: she is a lesbian. Up to thirty percent of female substance abusers are lesbians or bisexuals. The experiences of these women have been almost totally ignored.

*   *   *

Kit's Story

*We interviewed Kit on the moored boat of her close
friend. Kit is a tall, angular woman in her forties with a
short haircut, sparkling brown eyes and a wry smile. She
was wearing cut-off jeans and a windbreaker. She has
been clean for ten years.*

You may not think of me as your typical heroin addict because I
didn't prostitute myself and I didn't live on the street. But there are
a lot of junkies out there who are very very bright and well educated.
And I'll tell you one thing—the majority of drug abusers I've come
in contact with are highly spiritual beings who have been detoured
and are scared to death of their spirituality, or very very bright
people who have been told they're not. That's the kind of people I
know who have been into heavy drugs.

I was born in Detroit in 1945. As a child, I never got any of
those huggy, touchy kind of things. My mother is just a stone pillar
and my father is the same. I always got my love and support third
hand. Other people would tell me how much my parents loved me.

When I was three my parents moved to Arizona for my mom's
health. My dad gave up his business and was out of work for a long
time until he got a job as a welder with bridge builders. Every time
a bridge was completed, we'd move on.

When I was seven years old we went back to Detroit and moved
into the basement of my grandparents' house. We're talking cement
floors and no windows and a coal bin which was in use at the time.
We lived there for almost a year and it was a nightmare. From there
we moved to a one-bedroom apartment, my parents, myself, and
three brothers.

I pretty much grew up on the streets of inner-city Detroit. The
only guy I ever went with lived across the street and fell in love with
me when I was nine years old. Let's call him Jimmy. Jimmy was a
couple of years older. We went together when I was thirteen and
fourteen and when we broke up I tried to commit suicide. After
high school, I went to work for six months, saved my money, and

left for Southern California, where my older brother lived. Detroit was a nightmare and I was glad it was behind me.

I stayed with my brother for a couple of months and got a cushy job as an assistant to the artistic director in an ad agency. I made good money and was having fun. I had started drinking when I was fifteen, but now I could get into bars. I would go to lunch and have a couple of martinis and after work go out with friends and drink. That became a daily thing. I drank heavily for a long time. I just wanted to obliterate the world.

"He could provide for me and I could be a lady of leisure."

When I was about twenty-five I went back to Detroit on one of my annual hi-how-are-you-I'm-here-bye routines and I ran into Jimmy and we had a wild fling for the rest of the week I was there. Back in California I started getting letters from him. Next thing I knew, I found him on my doorstep and he lived with me for six highly charged, emotionally traumatic months. There was a lot of emotional craziness. What was wrong was that he was hooked on heroin and trying to kick. I hadn't even smoked marijuana at that point. I was a square about drugs so I knew nothing of the symptoms that I was seeing.

During these six months Jimmy turned me on to smoking weed and we dropped acid and mescaline a couple of times. Grass I loved. You know when you first start smoking grass you laugh and everything is fun. And there was no hangover. To me that was the greatest thing since knives and forks. You know, you get loaded and there's no hangover. I liked that a lot.

Jimmy got a job offer at a construction site in Australia and had ninety days before leaving. He said, "Marry me or I'm gone." That was just about the time I got the news my father was dying. For whatever reasons, I decided to marry Jimmy. Even today I'm not sure why. There was part of me that undoubtedly wanted to be with him, but marriage wasn't really on my agenda. I had been self-sufficient since I was seventeen. But he had the whole thing about wanting to take care of me, wanting to support me, that I shouldn't have to work. He could make good money. He could provide for me and I could just be a lady of leisure. As much as I hate to admit it at this stage in my life, I liked the idea of someone taking care of me. I had great plans for what I would do with my time. However, what I did with my time was not exactly what I had planned.

We got married and immediately left for Detroit. Within a week, Jimmy was back to using heroin. And on his home turf, he became real raving about everything. It was like, "This is the way it is. If you don't like it, tough sh—." He was very, very good to me in some areas and incredibly abusive in others. Like verbal abuse, running with the guys, not coming home. I felt totally helpless. I had no friends, no money, and I certainly couldn't borrow from my parents. After that first week, I began taking sleeping pills.

The first time I took a sleeping pill it was great. The experience was giddy. When you get past that initial drowziness, you get talkative, silly and you feel a kind of I-don't-give-a-damn attitude. Your body feels a little numbness, kind of like with alcohol. And if you're with other people who are feeling the same thing, it's funny and silly. You don't care about much. I immediately got into a regular habit of taking downs. I would get up in the morning, drink a bottle of wine, take a couple of downs, smoke a few joints, and then I would start my day. A bottle of wine turned into a daily routine. If we went out drinking, I would start with two or three shots of 150 proof rum and then I would start drinking. I could drink a tremendous amount for my size. I could drink just about anybody under the table. So for those first few months it was just downs and alcohol.

"I started wanting to use heroin to get back at him."

Australia fell through. So, for money, both of us dealt kilos of weed and we had a nice bankroll. Then we got into a lot of arguing and fighting. I knew I was unhappy and I didn't like what was going on, but it was almost as though I had just resolved to it. It was like I couldn't even see that there was another way to do things. It never crossed my mind that I could somehow pick up my life again and go back to California. Like it never dawned on me that I could do that.

Right after we moved out of my parents' basement, Jimmy promised he wasn't going to use anymore. I believed it. He always had an attitude of, "I'm not addicted, I can quit any time I want."

And I do have to hand it to him, he was one of the few junkies who could control his drug use. Which is more than I can say for myself. If he was starting to get real strung out, he'd get some Methadone and back off for three or four days. He thought he was a heroin user, not a heroin addict, and he really prided himself on that. And then he just started lying about being loaded. The interesting thing about people who use heroin is they think they can hide it. He'd sit there looking at me with his eyes as big as bowling balls, nodding out in the middle of a sentence, and swear up and down that he wasn't loaded.

There were some real bad fights between us, and more promises. One Sunday afternoon when I knew he had gone out to cop, I was laying for him. I waited for him to go into the head to fix. I waited just long enough. Just when he was getting ready to fix I forced my way into the bathroom. I was in a blind rage. I grabbed the spoon from him and tossed it across the room. You don't do that to a junkie. You know, I was asking to get pulverized. Which is what he did. He beat me real badly. Broke my nose and broke my jaw in two places. Took me to the hospital and literally dumped me.

I asked him for some phone money so I could call and have someone come and get me. He reached in his pocket to get some change and had five or six caps of heroin in his hand. He weeds through them and takes out a dime. I mean, talk about rubbing your nose in it! Then he takes off.

The next morning they wired my jaw. When I came out of surgery, he was there, his hair cut, his beard shaved and wearing nice clothes. He was crying and making promises: "I'll never hit you again, I'll never touch you again, I'll never use heroin again."

Part of the bargain was, not only would he not use any more heroin, but none of his buddies could come to the house to fix. Anytime someone wanted a fix they just came to our house. We had a shooting gallery going.

The next day, he went to work and my mother took me home from the hospital. I walk into the house. One of his junkie buddies is in my bed, there's a burnt screen on the bathroom sink, there's a trash can full of burnt matches and caps and a couple of ties on the door knobs. I made a scramble to pick up whatever was visible.

I remember feeling totally defeated. I had nowhere to go. I had no way out. I started wanting to use heroin, to get back at Jimmy for his lack of response to my begging him not to use. Jimmy didn't want me to use and no one would sell me any against his wishes. But I started running around with this girl who was going with a junkie. She got some heroin and we started fooling around just snorting it.

"I was strung out almost immediately."

Within the next couple of days Jimmy came home loaded and—you're going to love this, this is a great story—he decided that the only way he was going to stay clean was if he got me some dope and shot me up. He knew if he did that once, that would be it, because he didn't want me using dope and getting strung out. He'd never use again.

I was all for it. I wasn't having a great time with the nausea from snorting it. So, he went out and copped some dope and I fixed for the first time. And I loved it. You know, I had found what I wanted and that was it. After that first time, I never snorted again.

Those first few weeks were the first times that he and I had a communicative relationship. There was no more lying. There was no more hiding. There was a bond and a sense of well-being. You know. The family that fixes together stays together. We did our drugs together and we now had all the same friends. He turned me on to the connection so that I could go. And then money started getting tighter and tighter. Two arms are more expensive to feed than one. I was strung out almost immediately.

In the beginning I fixed just once a day, usually in the morning. Before too long it was twice a day, depending on how good the dope was. In those days you could get real loaded on a couple of dollars if you didn't have a habit going. If you were relatively clean, you could get loaded on five dollars easily. Once I got a bit of a habit going, then it was ten dollars, fifteen dollars. At that time a spoon was twenty-five dollars. Soon it was a couple of spoons a day, so I went to work.

I went to work for the creative director for these very posh architects who built big office buildings. I worked in the penthouse suite. And I was running into the head fixing!

Working there lasted about six months. I was really having a hard time dealing with it. I mean, I was either loaded or sick. I couldn't control my drug use. I was a pig about drugs. If I got any extra drugs, I didn't share it with Jimmy. I didn't even tell him I got it. I'd go down in the basement and fix up so he didn't know. I did a lot of laundry, you know what I mean? But it didn't take long for him to get my number and it scared him.

"I didn't consider myself addicted to any other drug."

I had been begging since we got to Detroit to go back to California. Finally in '72 he decided that things were out of hand, so we pack our little truck and take off for Arizona to stay with one of his buddies who had moved to Phoenix, an ex-user who had gotten married, had a baby, and was doing real well clean.

Within days of getting to our friends in Phoenix, we scored junk and started using and the friend was using after being clean over a year. We created absolute hell for that poor couple.

Using again really threw me into a tailspin. It's the first time I consciously knew that things were out of my control and I had to do something about what was going on. It was the first time since he beat me that I really hated him. It was the first time that all the hatred, pain, and anger came out. So I told him I had to get away for a few days and I took off for California.

In California I stayed with a woman I had met when I was seventeen. Her name was Mira and she was a nightclub entertainer. I had always had a thing for her, a crush on her, and we had remained friends through the years. For the first time I was in nice surroundings.

Jimmy followed me and begged me to come back. He couldn't understand how I could walk out on him. He never really understood the anger and hatred I was feeling. I have no idea where Jimmy is today or what he's doing. I heard three years ago from his mother that he was doing well, but I also heard from a niece who is a junkie that he was copping dope from her. So who knows?

I stayed with Mira about three months, went to work for an advertising agency in L.A., made good money, and stayed clean. Now when I say "clean," I mean clean of heroin. And when I say I got loaded, I mean heroin. I didn't consider myself addicted to any other drug. Other drugs were only substitutes for the state that I required on heroin. When I wasn't taking heroin I was taking downs—Tuinals and Seconals. It was either alcohol and downs or alcohol and tranquilizers. Valium, Librium, something. I was on something all the time.

"I mean by this point I'm desperate, I'm salivating."

After three months I moved into my own apartment. There was a woman working in the agency who I *knew* had access to drugs and I started thinking about getting loaded. Once you start thinking about it you can't let it go until you get loaded. You just can't. You know. It obsesses you. It owns you. So I approached her and it turned out she was going with a black guy who had connections. I told her I wanted to buy just a ten-dollar bag. She comes back the next day and she says, "He won't sell a ten-dollar bag, all he'll sell is a spoon." "Fine, I'll take a spoon." I gave her twenty-five dollars.

She comes back the next day and says, "All he'll sell is a gram," which was $125. Fine, I give her $125. Then she comes back and says, "He's changed his mind, all he'll sell me is a quarter." We're talking eight hundred dollars here. So I cough up eight hundred dollars. I mean by this point I'm desperate, I'm salivating. I had no other source in L.A. I had hung out at a couple of bars where I thought I could make a connection, and I was getting nowhere.

So anyway, she gets burned for the eight hundred dollars. She feels real bad about it and tells me that she knows another source. She'll put up four hundred dollars if I'll put up the other four hundred dollars. We could sell enough to get our money back. So she got it but it was cut so bad that it was already street quality so there's no way I can dilute it more. But I remembered that when I left Detroit it was pretty dry. They had some real bogus smack on the street. So, I decided, I'm going to go to Detroit with this and sell it all on a weekend, have a nice high and then come back and go to work.

I go to Detroit and it's saturated with the best dope they've ever had. Here I sit with my mediocre street sh—, staying with this guy who used to live upstairs from me and was kind of a yo-yo, not real swift. He was having a dealer come to test my dope and we didn't want the whole vial sitting there so he goes to the living room to stash it. He comes back, we fix, and it gets real warm so he turns on the air conditioning and all I hear is this clang, rattle, "Oh sh—!" He had hidden the vial in the air conditioner. I mean dope was flying through the air.

Needless to say I never made my money back on this deal, I never sold any of it. We spent the weekend staying nice and loaded. So I got strung out real bad again.

"When I left the hospital I began a life of crime."

Back in L.A., I bought a new house, bullsh—ted my way into a job making good money working for an animation studio and I got "clean" again. Then I get a letter from my mother saying that she's coming to visit. This really shocked me: the day before she arrived I started getting loaded and stayed loaded the whole time she was there. The whole time.

I got so strung out, I lost it. This job had me in way over my head and I ended up kind of having a nervous breakdown. I was on my way to work one day and I pulled off the freeway. I started crying, screaming. I couldn't relate to anything. I had just lost it.

I got myself to a telephone and called Mira. She took me to a psychiatrist who had me committed to a psychiatric hospital. The first day there they left me alone in the x-ray room. So I rummaged through the cupboards till I found a spinal needle this big around and used that and a plastic bottle from my contact lens solution to make a set of works. I got a hold of my junkie niece and she started bringing me drugs. I had a crater in my arm and I remember thinking, "Boy, you are crazy." But I would do anything to fix.

I spent two weeks basket weaving and playing arts and crafts. When I left the hospital I began a life of crime: forging checks, using bogus credit cards to make large purchases—televisions, stereos—then selling them. I had a network of people who were doing the same thing.

But I was so strung out I got careless and stupid and used my own credit cards and my own checks. I wasn't very smart in terms of crime.

So anyway, at Christmas I was living with this woman named Barbara in a gay relationship. She and I are coming home from getting some Christmas stuff and as I'm pulling into the driveway—it was just like in the movies: six cop cars with the spot lights on me, the red lights going, neighbors peeking out their windows. They get me spread-eagled against the car—the whole number.

They had me. I had credit cards on me and stolen property in my trunk. They take both of us in. I called someone and after one night I got out on bail. That was my one and only night in jail. Barbara's stuck there three days because I couldn't get the bail money for her. They ended up letting her go because they really had nothing to hold her on.

They charged me on seven counts of grand theft and forgery. They set bail which I was able to make on the arraignment. They assigned me to a probation officer who was a drug counselor kind of person. I had to go to him for counseling once a week until my case came up for trial.

"I can't get hold of my connection and I start to panic."

My drug counselor becomes my best friend and comes to my house to counsel me. He's going to help me. He's going to save me. He's going to make everything okay and take care of me. Before long, he starts buying my drugs for me and telling me he wants to marry me. This time I wasn't having any of it. Then he talked me into going to detox at a drug hospital to start preparing to go to court.

The hospital had two programs, a short-term ninety-day program and a long-term family program that lasted a year. After a week in the ninety-day program, I told them they could all f— themselves because I wasn't staying for their crazy games. I called my drug counselor to get twenty bucks and started using again. With my court date getting closer and closer I started cutting loose of the drugs a little bit. I had a real long running habit going at this point, so I'm able to let it go a little bit but not stop completely.

The weekend before I'm supposed to go to court, I can't get hold of my connection and I start to panic. How am I going to stand up in court going into full-fledged withdrawal? Then I remember that I had some Benadryl which has a real similar effect to heroin. I figure it'll save the day. So I open the caps and dissolve it in water. Usually I'd do a test run, but I was so desperate I just ran the whole six capsules. As soon as it started going up my arm I knew I was in trouble. It felt like my arm was going to explode. I was standing in front of the mirror and as I look into it my feeling was that I was watching myself die. My skin turned grey. The color of my eyes completely disappeared. My pupils went—woong. Everything got totally distorted and I started losing consciousness. I was able to get to the phone to call my drug counselor, who called an ambulance. My vital signs were real bad.

They took me to the state hospital and classified me as an attempted suicide. In the State of California if you're an attempted suicide it's a mandatory seventy-two-hour observation in a mental ward. All I can grasp is that the hospital I'm in, aside from being a cracker factory, is the mother drug program to the one that I had just been in, the one where they do the long-term treatment. I think, "I'm a drug addict so they put me in the drug program. Where else would they take me?"

They do this lightweight interview and shoot me up with Thorazine. The next day I wake up I'm in a six- or eight-bed ward. I go out of the room and walk down the hall to the nurses' station thinking, "Ah-ha, I'll just go get me some Methadone or something." I stood in the doorway and asked if I could have some Methadone. They all looked at me as if I were crazy and told me to go on about my business. So I went back to my room and found the door locked. An attendant comes by and tells me: "All the rooms are locked until four o'clock." I said, "But I was just in there." He said, "Go down in the day room."

"I was facing ten years in the state penitentiary."

The day room was my first indication that I was in a locked mental ward. Did you see *One Flew Over the Cuckoo's Nest*? Well, that's what it was. These were crazies. Of the entire ward of about thirty women, I found two I could hold any kind of a conversation with and one of them was a little shaky. I mean we're talking righteous Looney Tunes here. I was on that ward for three days.

If you approach a doctor or a nurse and tell them you are not crazy, they immediately know you are crazy and you're right where you belong. When a doctor comes on the unit, all these people literally get on the floor and pull on his coat. And if you make any waves in a state hospital, you get Thorazine immediately. Half the people on that ward walked around with what they call the Thorazine shuffle: out of it.

Monday morning a social worker came on the floor and I pulled her aside and told her what was going on. She believed me and made a couple of phone calls and found, yes, I was due in court, that a bench warrant had been issued, that I was in deep trouble, and belonged in a drug unit. So they got hold of my drug counselor who got hold of my attorney who called the judge who pulled the bench warrant so that I would go directly to the drug program—the long-term program—which really thrilled me no end.

So I committed myself to the long-term program on April 10th, 1974. I went there only because I was facing trial. I had no intention of giving up drugs. The only thing that kept me there was the fact that I was facing ten years in the state penitentiary. I was in treatment for nine months. During those nine months I didn't use at all.

The program I was in, like most such programs, was made up primarily of men and run by men who came directly out of the penal system. Most were there either for drug-related murders or dealing. The few women who came were heavy cases who were court committed. It was: either you're in a drug program or you're in prison. There was no "Well if you don't stay we'll give you another chance."

In those days there were very few restrictions on what drug programs could do. They shaved our heads. We scrubbed toilets with toothbrushes. We were allowed an average, and I'm not exaggerating, of two hours' sleep a night. Once a week we'd get a full night's sleep.

The whole purpose was to keep your defenses down so they could get to the core of what was going on. It was an offshoot of Synanon and they played Synanon games. When the federal government finally stepped in, it changed a lot of ways the long-term treatment programs were handled. But this program was run by dope fiends and people who had spent most of their lives in prison—people full of so much hate, anger, and pain that they spent their time dumping it on whoever they could. And it was a situation where women got dumped on continuously.

"There were a lot of cruel and devastating things."

When I went into the program, I was in what they called the candidacy. I wore baby clothes. I carried baby toys. I was never allowed to look a family member in the eye. If a family member walked down the hall I had to put my nose against the wall. After candidacy, you'd become a family member and after that you went on staff. Then you became an elder which means you're in charge of the whole house.

Here's a typical kind of a week in the first two phases of the program. Beginning in the morning, it's clean-up. White glove clean-up. Literally, somebody came around with a white glove. They would plant dirt. They would find bogus things to get on your case about that would get you disciplined. Then, therapies running from eight in the morning until nine at night, or later if there are things they want to deal with.

What they tried to do was create petty situations that would cause you to behave the way you would on the street if someone pissed you off, if someone crossed you or hurt your feelings. Because petty things are no longer petty when you have nothing else to relate them to. When you're in that confined situation, somebody stealing a piece of cake out of the kitchen in the middle of the night is no different than breaking into the local drugstore and taking drugs.

They spent a great deal of energy purposely making people angry to make them get to their pain. And they attempted to break the snitch code. Everyone had to tell on everyone else, and learn to trust that that person wouldn't kill them. So there were a lot of processes going on and a lot of very constructive therapies.

The good counselors attempted to put you back together when it was over, but there were a lot of cruel and devastating things that happened. They woke me up at all hours of the night and kept me up, scrubbing with a toothbrush while I was dressed in things that made it difficult to move: socks on my hands, a bag on my head, tied to somebody else, left and right legs tied together.

Then two things happened that changed my life as far as the program was concerned.

"I realized I was literally fighting for my life."

One night, they got us up and they had brought trash from detox. I mean we're talking trash—coffee grounds mixed with cigarette butts. They threw it all over the floor and hallway. Then they stood us, nose and toes to the wall for probably two hours. And the whole time they're calling me every motherf—ing thing they can think of. Then they got us on our hands and knees to clean the floor. They send us back to bed, and twenty minutes later they do it again. They did it four times. And we're talking scrubbing and waxing on our hands and knees. The last time, they put water down on the floor and made us crawl on our bellies. At that point, I was so angry and frustrated I wanted to kill. And I realized for the first time I was literally fighting for my life. I knew that if I could put up with this kind of sh— and abuse I could survive on the street. There was no doubt in my mind that I could make it on the street. And it was the first time I seriously considered that I could make it without drugs.

The second thing was, when I came into the program I knew I'd have no contact with the outside world. No radio, no TV, no letters, no phone calls. But I had things that needed to be taken care of—a dog that was very precious to me, a house and a car. So I gave power of attorney to my drug counselor who had gone to work for the hospital I was in. He was going to live in the house, make the payments, and take care of my dog.

Well, first of all, he was on speed. He just took the money and let my house go into foreclosure. He had a rock band living there with him and they pretty much wrecked everything that was in it. Then he moved out.

And . . . this is very hard for me to talk about. [Pauses, crying] You'll have to wait a minute. Oh, God. [Pause] He had left my dog Sammy in the house, tied up. He just locked him up in the house and let him die. And when he was confronted about it, this son-of-a-bitch had the f—ing balls to look me in the eye and tell me, not only did he let him die but he put him in the garbage and let them take him away.

That was the major turning point. The only way I could accept and deal with what happened was to know that Sammy had given up his life for me and I would have to do something about it. I had to make it so he didn't die for nothing. That's when I really started to fight back.

"They could take the program and shove it."

I was in the program for nine months. I was the first female to have gotten that far. They decided to make me the first woman elder. You have to understand I was not the person I am today. I was crazy. I was mean. I was vicious. I hated the world. I mean, don't even look at me cross-eyed, motherf—er. That's where I was at. I treated people under me certainly no better than I had been treated. I was the one who woke them up in the middle of the night. I was the one who stood them on the wall all day long.

Then they put me back to candidacy. It wasn't the first time they did something like that. They did it to test me and break me down. They left me there for four weeks, which was unheard of. And I decided that as soon as they moved me back up, I was gone. They could take the program and shove it. And if I went to jail, I went to jail.

They brought me back up and the next day I left. I was real scared because I left out of pride, ego, anger, and the whole f—-you attitude. Once I was on the street, I didn't know what I was going to do. My case was still pending, and the one criterion to keep me out of prison was that I complete the program. I didn't know what was going to happen to me.

My attorney really went to bat for me. When we went to court, the judge says I should be committed for ninety days' observation in a state institution. My attorney jumps up, "But your Honor, she just spent nine months!" So they go back and forth for a couple of minutes and finally the judge says, "I'm going to put this case off for another thirty days." And he looks at me and says, "If you're working within thirty days, and you're clean, and you haven't gotten into any trouble, then we'll decide your fate."

Thirty days later I went back to court. I had a job restoring and selling sports cars. The judge found me guilty and sentenced me to ten years in the state penitentiary. I almost fainted. But he suspended the sentence and put me on five years' probation. The terms of my probation were that I be tested for drugs, that I stay out of trouble and pay back nine thousand dollars. And if I broke any term of my probation, my sentence would go into effect immediately.

I gulped, thanked him very much, left the courtroom, and reported to Probation.

"It was the final battle with heroin."

When I came out of treatment, roughly March of 1975, I was clean for about three months and then I started drinking for two or three months. I started using again. I used three times. But each time I got so violently sick that the third time I finally realized that God was saying, "Hey, this is it. You want to die? Fine. Here. Knock yourself out."

Cold turkey on heroin is no big deal. It hurts and it's painful and you're sure you're dead but you're not going to die. It's not like coming off Valium or some of the other sleeping pills—which you can die from. That's not true of heroin. What I did experience in the long term was withdrawal symptoms like sweats, depression, nausea, and a feeling in my back and shoulders like a nerve reaction. It's crawling, you just feel horrible. The biggest thing was sweats and nerves. I experienced those things well up to a year after I stopped taking drugs.

I was really able to totally let go of heroin three years ago. My junkie niece called and asked if I would go to court with her. So I did. Like anyone who used drugs or alcohol, I couldn't be around someone who uses without thinking about it. So the whole time we were in court I was thinking about it. And then I went back to her house and purposefully started hanging out, knowing she was getting ready to cop, battling with myself, "Do I want to do this or not?" Back and forth. Back and forth. Yes. No. Yes. No. She finally got some dope. I stayed while she fixed, still debating whether or not I was going to ask her if I could have some. I didn't know what I was going to do. But I knew I wanted it.

Finally I got up the nerve to walk away. It was the final battle with heroin, the battle of good and evil. And I knew I had won. And that was it.

"For the first time, I didn't have that emptiness inside."

I became friendly with a couple who knew I was living a gay lifestyle. They introduced me to a woman who wanted to get involved with another woman. She owned a film and video company with offices in L.A. and New York. I started seeing her from time to time when she was in L.A. She hired me, trained me for six months, and drove me to New York to take over her New York office. I became vice president of sales for the East Coast. I did very well. I made good money. I really established myself.

Shortly after I got to New York I went into therapy and my whole life turned completely around. I got into health. I got into exercise. I became a vegetarian and I had no more desire to smoke dope or drink alcohol. So that changed my lifestyle. Suddenly I'm not a barfly.

And while I had proved to myself that I could be successful and make a lot of money, I found out that's not what I really want. I saved my money, quit my job, went to Woodstock, and wrote. And I discovered photography. That was what got me past my fear of creating and that was when I decided that my life had to revolve around creativity.

When I found the camera, that was it. I decided to come back to California, which was in '81. A friend of mine is a director and she got me some jobs in film production. For the first time, I didn't have that emptiness inside.

I like myself as a person. I recognize my oneness with God. I know people like me and I know my past doesn't make any difference. It's like coming back home. It's recognizing who I am, and who I am is a form of God.

That's it. That's my whole story.

12

The Pattern of Experience

When we started writing this book, we made every effort to choose women whose stories would represent a cross section of lifestyles. We spoke to rich and poor, young and old, heterosexual and lesbian, white and black, professional and homemaker. We think this effort has been worth it. The life story of an inner-city heroin addict gives us a picture of the chemically dependent woman that we could not possibly get from a to-the-manor-born cocaine abuser, and vice versa.

But in rereading these stories we see something even more significant: despite age, race, social set, sexual orientation, or drug of choice, these women, and millions like them, have shared critical experiences, stretching from childhood through recovery. These experiences deepened our awareness that chemically dependent men and women live in fundamentally different cultures.[1]

Men's experience has always formed the basis of our understanding of substance abuse—what impact it has on the individual, the family, and society. As recently as a decade ago, a search of the literature uncovered only fifty articles devoted to chemically dependent women, among thousands devoted to men.[2] If women's experience didn't fit the accepted paradigm of substance abuse, or if women didn't benefit from treatment as much as men, it was concluded that they were "less normal" than men.[3] They were the round pegs which didn't fit the square holes.

The challenges chemically dependent and recovering women confront have as much to do with their being women as with their being addicts. As a user a woman is more ostracized than a man.[4] If she seeks medical help, she runs a greater risk of being tranquilized and untreated than a man. If she looks for help in a treatment program, there is a good possibility she will wind up in a male-oriented and male-staffed treatment facility where her needs are unrecognized or simply ignored.[5,6] In some treatment centers, she might even be propositioned by male staff members and have little choice but to acquiesce.[7]

In the male-oriented view, the chemically dependent person is a sick individual, suffering from a physical, emotional, and psychological disease.[8] This model has served us well in blunting the stigma of addiction. And recent research—with men—does indeed indicate a genetic factor in alcoholism. But the great majority of chemically dependent women cite difficult life events as precipitating factors in their drug use. Typically, a woman uses chemicals to reduce stress and to cope with her life, and to anesthetize her painful, negative feelings. If we view the chemically dependent woman as a victim of the very same disease that strikes men, we ignore the unique situational stresses and cultural pressures that impact her—and all women.[9]

The similarities of experience we and others have found in female chemical abuse and recovery interface with wide-ranging social and political issues, beginning at birth and ending on the highest level of personal experience. Among them are:

- Most of the recovering women we talked to felt out of place and unhappy as children.[10]

- More than half of all chemically dependent women are survivors of childhood incest or molestation.

- Women feel lower self-esteem before, during, and after chemical dependency than men do.

- Nearly half of all chemically dependent women have been battered or raped. Most have been abused emotionally.[11]

- After repeated abuse, women learn to be helpless and feel powerless over their lives.

- Women need to develop assertiveness skills.

- The needs of chemically dependent minority women have been largely ignored.

- Lesbians have higher rates of alcoholism and suffer a double stigma in recovery.

- Women addicts suffer greater social stigma than men addicts and feel greater shame about their drug abuse.

- Women hide their addiction more than men.

- Women experience greater isolation and abandonment than men.

- Drug abuse progresses more rapidly and more destructively in women than in men.

- Many women who enter treatment need childcare.

- Most women who enter treatment need job skills.

Feeling different

Ann Wilson Schaef observes that women are born "tainted" with the Original Sin of Being Born Female and no amount of good work will absolve them.[12] In our survey of nearly one hundred recovering women, more than ninety percent felt out of place and unhappy as children. One recovering alcoholic said, "I always felt as though the mother ship had left and I was stranded on an alien planet."

Most women remembered their parents being emotionally cold and unapproachable. Nanci said, "I remember as a kid sitting on my bed saying, 'Why doesn't daddy love me? He doesn't love me. He doesn't hold me. He doesn't kiss me.' " Laura remembered, "My mother would say, 'Gee, I love you,' and somehow at the same time she was pinching me real bad and I'd think, 'Why does it hurt?' " Kit said, "My father is just a stone pillar and my mother is the same."

Incest and molestation

A surprisingly large percentage of women report being survivors of incest, as Melanie did. While reports of child sexual abuse in day-care centers and schools make the front pages with increasing regularity, sexual abuse among family members is still shrouded in silence and denial. Fifty years ago, incest was considered a one-in-a-million occurrence.[13] Even as late as the seventies no more than five thousand children a year were believed to be victims.[14] We now know better: current estimates are that 250,000 children are sexually molested in their homes each year; seventy-five percent of these violations are between fathers and daughters.[15]

Surveys of female sexual abuse both in and out of the family come to even more alarming conclusions: up to one-third of *all* women have been victims of childhood sexual molestation. Yet nearly *two-thirds* of the women in some drug treatment centers have been molested before the age of fourteen, and nearly half have been victims of incest.[16-18] Female incest victims have drug abuse rates seven times higher than nonvictimized females.[19]

The immediate effects of sexual molestation on its victims can be devastating—anger, fear, sleep and eating problems, confusion, isolation, and shame are common. The naive belief that time heals these wounds is part of the overall minimization and denial of the molestation experience.[20] Decades after the violations have stopped, many women continue to react with impaired emotionality, sexual dysfunctions, anxiety, depression, guilt, mistrust, and poor self-image—disorders that many experts agree often set the stage for drug abuse.[21,22]

But sexual abuse of young girls does more than predispose them to drug and alcohol abuse. It is often a link in a chain of abuse that is lifelong or even intergenerational. Many girls who are molested do not develop the skills necessary to care for and protect themselves or their children.

- More than one-third of women who are multiply raped are survivors of incest.[23]

- Nearly two-thirds of incest victims suffer major depression in adult life; more than one-third attempt suicide.[24]

- Incest survivors are more likely to come from violent homes and are likely to tolerate an abusive husband.[25]

- The sexual problems incest survivors experience in their own marriages—inability to experience orgasm, or even sexual arousal, and subsequent reluctance to have sex—often create a sequence of events that leads to the molestation of their own daughters. Mothers of abused children are eight times more likely to report an experience of incest than mothers of nonabused children.[26]

- And finally, survivors of sexual abuse often grow up regarding themselves and other women with contempt. They avoid close and nurturing relationships with other women and often have no one to turn to in times of crisis.[27]

Thus, for a majority of female drug abusers, establishing fully sober lives—repairing faulty self-esteem, accepting the healing fellowship of other women, relating to men as equals—means dealing with all the issues surrounding childhood sexual trauma. As with Melanie, overcoming the effects of childhood molestation and getting clean sometimes go hand in hand. But in counseling women molested as children we have come to believe that a recovering woman needs to feel stabilized in her sobriety before attempting the painful, healing journey back to the past. She needs to know, too, that this journey can be made easier with the help and guidance of other survivors of incest who have explored the depth of their pain and have been restored.[28]

Self-esteem

The lower self-esteem of drug dependent women compared to drug-dependent men, and the lower expectations they have for their lives, comes out of their social milieu.[29] Churches, schools, and the media are permeated with powerful and positive male role models while women are peripherally or negatively presented. The study of history is the study of the exploits of men. George Washington forges a nation while Betsy Ross sews a flag.

The times may be changing for women, but the traditional undervaluation of female contributions to society—economically and status-wise—continues to have an enormous negative impact on how women feel about themselves. This is the groundwork for the seriously impaired self-esteem typically found in women. When authors Linda Tschirhart Sanford and Mary Ellen Donovan asked women to tell their stories, they were told by many, "Oh, you don't want to bother with me." When they asked women to come up with one thing they like about themselves, most had difficulty in answering with anything more profound than, "I like my teeth." Sanford and Donovan conclude that, despite women's presenting themselves "more proudly and confidently in public, in the privacy of their own minds too few . . . consider themselves truly valuable." They "habitually downgrade their own worth."[30]

Family therapist Judy Saalinger, who has worked with over a hundred chemically dependent women, told us, "Women feel that their self is their body and what they put on their body and how their skin looks and how their teeth look and what they wear—jewelry, cars, everything—those things become primary as to who they are rather than defining themselves from their inner self. They have an empty self."

And here, we feel, is an essential difference between the tasks of chemically dependent men and women in recovery. While for recovering men it is important to *restore* their sense of self and self-esteem, for recovering women it is critical to *create* a sense of self and self-esteem.

Battering and marital rape

Low self-esteem leads an enormous number of women into relationships where they are the underdogs. Nonaddicted as well as chemically dependent women get into abusive relationships, but the latter report more severe and longer-lasting abuse.[31] Three-quarters of the women we spoke to said they had been physically and/or emotionally abused by men, most of them repeatedly.

Until fairly recently, domestic violence against women was dismissed as a private matter and a man's prerogative. Often, the victim herself was blamed—"She had it coming," "She deserved it," "She must have provoked it," and so on. Clearly, attitudes have changed considerably, yet wife battering remains perhaps the most widespread of all crimes, and the most underreported. *Half* of all American wives experience some form of physical abuse from their husbands, yet as few as *one-third of one percent* of batterings come to the attention of legal authorities.[32,33]

The reasons men batter are varied, but substance abuse is primary among them—most batterers have clear drug or alcohol problems.[34] Surprisingly, one study of battered wives found that nearly three-quarters of *them* were frequent drinkers.[35] Whether or not a woman becomes a substance abuser before or because of physical violence is still a question for study. But there is little doubt that the same psychological conditions that predispose a woman to alcohol and drug dependence also predispose her to tolerate an abusive partner: she is more likely to come from an abusive home, she suffers low self-esteem, and she tends to feel isolated.[36]

This sense of isolation is especially strong for middle-class women, for whom battering is surrounded with the same sense of shame and guilt of chemical dependency itself. Laura's story epitomized their experience—don't talk about the abuse, because even if you do, no one will believe you.

Laura was also raped by her husband. Marital rape is a term that even today many people see as a contradiction. In fact, it is considered a crime in only eleven states. To the women who are victims, it is rape nonetheless, and can lead to increased alcohol and drug use, severe depression, and suicide.[37,38] Marital rape occurs in about one out of ten marriages, but it is committed in half of all battering relationships, which means that battered women have up to five times more risk of being raped by their husbands as nonbattered women.[39,40]

The best reaction for the battered wife, according to some experts, is to call the police and do everything necessary to get the batterer arrested. On average, men who are arrested are dramatically less likely to batter again.[41] But those few women who finally do press charges have been battered, on average, more than thirty times.[42]

Learned helplessness

Battered women stay with their abusive partners not only because of the debilitating effects of their alcohol or drugs, but because, with repeated abuse, they eventually *learn to be helpless*.[43] These women feel unable to stop what is happening to them and see no alternatives to staying where they are. They suffer from a depressing sense of powerlessness over their own lives. Kit, our heroin addict, recalled, "It was like I couldn't even see that there was another way to live. It almost never crossed my mind that I could . . . pick up my life again." A speed addict told us, "I was such a nothing, I couldn't even ask for help." Because chemically dependent women feel they don't deserve help, or that it won't make a difference, they have not sought treatment in anywhere near the same proportion as men.[44]

In recovery, these survivors of helplessness need relationships founded on respect and equality, and interaction with female counselors and therapists who can offer positive female role models. They need experiences which empower them in ways which men routinely take for granted. Historically, when women have asserted themselves, the fruits of their action were often subtly stolen from them. Women fought for the right to vote for seventy years; yet, according to the popular wisdom, they were "given" the vote.

Assertiveness

Lack of assertiveness is pandemic among women and is as critically related to female substance abuse as it is to mental health in general.[45] From early infancy, males are trained to be independent and presented with aggressive and powerful role models. These inculcated traits, they are taught, are the very traits society values. The ideal female roles are ones of passivity, nurturance, dependence, and service to others, traits which society undervalues.

Because males have abrogated as "masculine" those traits that both sexes need to feel good about themselves and to function autonomously in the world—including forcefulness, self-reliance, and assertiveness—women need to discover these "masculine" traits in themselves.[46]

Assertiveness training has been called one of the most powerful tools for overcoming some of the harmful effects of sex-role socialization—helplessness, passivity, and dependency.[47] But female assertiveness training cannot simply be grafted onto a male-oriented, male-staffed treatment model and still be effective. In mixed gender therapy groups women are generally outnumbered and typically feel a lack of support, while males bond together and jockey for dominance.[48] If sobriety is to be viable, recovering women need to overcome their learned fear and anxiety of assertive behavior.[49]

Minority women

In the chemical dependency treatment field there is probably no more neglected population than chemically dependent minority women. They have been called the "invisible" addicts because so few appear at treatment centers or Twelve-Step meetings. Most minority women live within a cultural system so closed, and a socioeconomic level so low, their problems cannot even be identified, much less treated.[50] In research, they have been neglected: few studies on Hispanics mention women, and studies of Asian-American women are nonexistent.

Yet in some ways minority women suffer more effects of substance abuse than any other group. Rates of cirrhosis of the liver among black women is more than six times the rate for white women.[51] More than twice as many black women die from liver disease as white women.[52] Among blacks who drink, twice as many women as men report alcohol-related health problems.[53]

The drinking habits of black women and white women differ dramatically. Research in the last decade has shown that, on the one hand, more black women abstain totally, and on the other, more black women—three times as many—engage in heavy drinking.[54] Alcohol-related deaths among white women in the ten years between 1964 and 1974 rose thirty-six percent; deaths among nonwhite women, mostly black, rose seventy-one percent.[55] Black alcoholic women were more frequently hospitalized and had more arrests than white women—fifty percent to seventeen percent—and had a history of more school problems.[56] In 1983, one out of five women who died of drug abuse was black.[57]

The particular stresses on the native American woman—ethnic prejudice, impaired health, marginal economic existence, high unemployment, rampant alcoholism among the men in her family, and control by non-Indian social agencies of her family's and community's life—are powerful contributing factors to their high rates of substance abuse.[58] Wanda Frogg, director of the North American Indian Women's Council on Chemical Dependency, estimates that sixty percent of native American women are alcoholic.[59] One in every four deaths among Indian women is caused by alcoholic cirrhosis—a rate *thirty-seven* times higher than the rate among white women.[60]

Despite the alarming rates of chemical dependency among minority women, in 1976 they made up only twenty percent of the clientele of all federally-supported native American programs, seventeen percent of patients in black programs, and a bare eight percent in Hispanic programs.[61]

Feelings of shame, family denial, and a reluctance to interact with the white, middle-class, male power structure often keep native American and Hispanic women from getting the treatment they need. The director of the Office on Alcoholism for the state of California commented that if "other women [are] known as closet alcoholics . . . the Spanish-speaking woman is in the basement."[62] One professional working with native American women wrote, "even though we can get them to admit they are alcoholics, it is very difficult for them to learn to forgive themselves."[63]

The problems of cultural stigma and denial are compounded by treatment providers who slate their services to whites, in white neighborhoods, with white staffs, with a white male focus and white male cultural values. It is small wonder that minority women have shunned these services.[64]

Once they are in treatment, however, minority women contribute enormously and uniquely. Often, they are more comfortable in expressing anger, in being assertive, and in bonding with other women. Black female addicts show self-esteem rates twice as high as white women in treatment and have a higher success rate.[65] Because black women experience less crippling shame and are less concerned than white women about questions of "respectability," they are excellent role models.[66] And although three times as many black female heroin addicts as white female heroin addicts support themselves as prostitutes, overall, the great majority of black female addicts have high self-concepts.[67]

Lesbians

Lesbians have been called a double minority, and suffer status reduction both as women and as gays.[68] Lesbians have higher rates of alcoholism than heterosexual women—nearly six times higher according to some studies—and are more likely to use nonprescription drugs. One-third of all gays are alcoholic or at risk for alcoholism.[69,70] Several researchers point to the central role of the gay bar in lesbian social life as an important reason for this high rate. According to Brenda Underhill, Executive Director of the Alcoholism Center for Women in Los Angeles, the gay bar "may be the only place a lesbian feels she can socialize and be open about her sexuality. Helping her reorient her social life to chemical-free environments is . . . a major issue in recovery."

Homosexuality is no longer considered a mental illness, but a tendency to regard lesbians as "sick" still exists, both among health care professionals and among those lesbians who have internalized the homophobia of the culture and have turned it against themselves. In many treatment centers the stigma of homosexuality appears to be applied more severely to females.[71] In fact, lesbians are more likely to leave treatment midstream because of harsher discrimination stemming from treatment staffs' homophobic reactions.[72]

Despite the fact that homosexuality is reported much more often among women addicts than men addicts—some studies show that at least one-third of all female addicts are either bisexual or homosexual—homoemotional identity remains an issue usually not attended to in recovery because treatment staffs are not sufficiently sensitive to lesbians, and many lesbians are understandably reluctant to talk about lesbian issues in mixed groups.[73,74] But when lesbian addicts were treated in their own group at the Betty Ford Center, they *had the highest recovery rate* for any group ever treated there.[75] In fact, lesbians in treatment have "more self-confidence" than heterosexual women and higher levels of self-esteem than a random sample of college women.[76,77] Authors Dana Finnegan and Emily B. McNally caution that most studies of lesbians involve women who, in identifying themselves as lesbians, have already integrated their sexuality into their identity and consequently enjoy a higher self-concept. Such high levels of self-esteem would not be found among the vast majority of closeted lesbians who are frightened, confused, and terrified of being discovered.[78] And with good reason, since a woman stands to lose her most important support systems—her job, her family, and the custody of her children.[79]

Lesbianism often surfaces with new urgency and meaning in recovery. A woman may find herself asking questions like, "Now that I'm clean and sober, am I really a lesbian?" Or, "Will I continue to be a lesbian?" Or, "Now that I'm clean and sober should I come out of the closet?" Or, "Must I label myself?" Or, "Am I willing to label myself?" Such questions are bound to engage the recovering woman—gay, straight, or bisexual—as she explores her emotional and sexual identity, and allows it to blossom.

Stigmatization

Connecting with others is critical for the recovering woman. Ninety-five percent of the one hundred women we informally surveyed said they felt isolated during their substance abuse. Unlike men—who may have friends, drinking buddies, and co-workers with whom they socialize even in the most progressed stages of addiction—women substance abusers are more stigmatized, and more often use drugs at home or alone.[80]

The greater stigmatization of female addicts causes them to deny their dependency and hide their drugs. Seventy-five percent of the women we interviewed hid their drugs—in attics, under sinks, in car trunks, or safe-deposit boxes. Others patronized several different dealers, doctors, or liquor stores so one knew how much they were using. The chemically dependent woman comes to believe that, by hiding the drugs, she can conceal the effects of the drugs. This denial is reinforced and legitimized by the "social myopia" of family, friends, and doctors. But inevitably, drugs take their toll—on her and on her relationships.

Abandonment and isolation

Wives of chemically dependent men generally stick by their husbands and support their recovery.[81,82] But women are more often abandoned, or more likely to have partners who themselves use drugs and are therefore ambivalent about their spouses' recovery.[83] Thus, a woman commonly finds herself in fearful isolation at the very time she is "hitting bottom" and most needs the support of family and friends.

Hitting bottom harder

Abandonment is one reason why hitting bottom is a more painful and wrenching experience for women. Another is that drug abuse progresses more rapidly and with more serious consequences in women than in men. More female alcoholics develop hepatatis, more begin their recovery with an accompanying illness, or with acute complications such as confusion or suicide attempts.[84] Jill, referring to her estranged alcoholic husband, told us, "In the three years we hadn't seen each other, his drinking had stayed the same. He was still what you call a 'functioning alcoholic.' He could function fine at work, be the first one out to the bar at the office, start drinking, get pretty high by the time he got home, go to bed, and do the same thing *ad infinitum*. And maintain. Whereas I had started going down like a rock."

Childcare needs

Abandoned by friends and spouses, a large majority of women nonetheless embark on recovery with child-rearing responsibilities; yet most communities woefully ignore their needs.[85-88] Lack of adequate childcare programs is a dilemma for nonaddicted women; it is a catastrophe for recovering women. It is part of our collective mindset that somehow substance abusing females—and their children—should fend for themselves. We are the only industrialized nation without a comprehensive childcare program.

In treatment programs the chemically dependent woman is often needlessly handicapped and placed in a cruel double bind. On the one hand she is expected to adhere to the program's rigorous schedule; on the other hand she is expected to continue to care for her children. If she brings her child to treatment, she is bothered by constant interruptions and receives ineffective treatment.[89] If she leaves her child with inadequate care, she is being neglectful.

Job skill needs

Recovering women frequently find themselves without money, medical insurance, job skills, job availability, or even a place to live. They have only themselves; in the words of black author Chaney Allen, they are "standing in the middle of everything they own." This predicament cries out for special attention. Only a tiny minority of women enter treatment programs with a history of continuous employment, and more than a third have had no employment for years.[90] One study of twenty-five treatment programs serving recovering women found that two-thirds of the clients received no vocational counseling.[91]

Both recovering men and women consider a lack of money their
most serious problem. The applied solution is often to give men
vocation skill training, while offering women social skill training.[92]
Clearly, the same devaluation of female skills that operates in the
society at large is reflected in many treatment programs. A significantly greater number of recovering men than recovering women are
referred for job placement.[93] Upon discharge from treatment, more
than three-quarters of female clients remain unemployed.[94]

Growing awareness

In trying to understand the source of the problem of female drug
abuse, we have been forced to confront a host of deeper ills that
plague us. Our culture, Karen Horney wrote, is a male culture, not
favorable to the unfolding of a woman's individuality. Low self-
esteem, abuse, stigmatization, abandonment, isolation, and unemployment—this commonality of experience that we have seen in the
ten stories in this book—are the legacy of our society's profound
sexism. What is new is the willingness of so many women to speak
up. And the willingness of so many to listen. Just as overcoming
denial is the first step an individual takes toward recovery, women's
growing awareness of the full scope of their predicament is surely
the most powerful catalyst of change.

But awareness is only the first step. Newly recovering women
need enlightened professionals familiar with the burdens women
carry from a lifetime of addiction compounded by disenfranchise-
ment. We have come to see that the path of women in recovery must
be a process of *empowerment* that gives them the perspective, the
skills, and availability of services which enable them to realize their
human potential on a parity with men. Women have the right to the
delivery of chemical dependency services specifically designed for
them.

As chemical dependency counselors working in hospital settings,
we have seen how, in the presence of male staffers, women often
continue the behavior they have been taught men respond to—those
typically "feminine" traits like hysteria, coyness, and girlish incom-
petence—behavior that doesn't cut it in recovery. How often have

where the few women patients sat sullen, or sniped at each other, or flirted with male patients, but otherwise isolated themselves—while the men dealt with their issues. At one such hospital in-patient program, when the patient population was particularly high, the patients would be split into separate men's and women's groups. Then the women broke loose and sparks flew. The women began to explore their feelings toward each other and toward women in general. They began to validate each other and themselves, not as cute and attractive as men validated them, but for their human qualities and shared experience. They began, often for the first time in their lives, to form significant, growth-oriented bonds with other women. They brought up their experiences with incest, abuse, battering, sexual promiscuity and orientation; they spoke of their shame and abandonment, their fears about trust and intimacy, mothering, making money, and what it was like to grow up in homes where male siblings got all the prizes. Not one of these was a topic they could feel safe about discussing in a mixed group. Yet these were the issues that held the key to their bondage or freedom.

Spiritual awakening

Carl Jung labelled alcoholism and, by implication, drug addiction, a disease of the spirit. In 1961 he wrote to Bill Wilson, co-founder of AA, that the craving for alcohol "was the equivalent on a low level of the spiritual thirst for our being for wholeness, expressed in medieval language: the union with God." It would be extremely short-sighted to look at this "thirst" as a mere side effect of sobriety. Rather, a spiritual awakening may be *essential* to recovery. As Carl Jung went on to say, alcohol in Latin is *spiritus*, the very word we use for the highest religious experience. Therefore, he concluded, *spirits* can only be fought with *spirit*.[95]

Every recovering woman we spoke with in the course of writing this book had experienced a spiritual awakening, a belief in God, or a higher power, and started living with hope.

In the case of some women, this spiritual awakening came as faith that God was guiding them through the difficult times: "I was terrified of going to the market and terrified of the laundromat. The choices were just overwhelming to me . . . . So . . . I'd say things

like, 'Okay, God, you decide which cereal and I'll get it.' I trusted
that God was giving me the right stuff. That's how God proved
himself to me, all those little silly things of surviving the day.''

For Jill this awakening came as a reconnection with other
people and unfolded at her first AA meeting: ''That's where I first
got that magic hope. I just grabbed onto that with both hands . . .
When everybody held hands . . . I started to cry . . . because I felt
like I had come home.''

And, finally, for some women, spiritual awakening came as an
intimation that the despair and darkness of their lives could somehow
end. We recall Melanie, alone in a hospital room, in the throes of a
violent withdrawal: ''All I could think of was the bad things. I
thought—'Jeepers, I've woken up in rubber rooms. I've been in
cracker factories. My whole life has been about abuse . . .' And I
realized that I was having some really negative kind of thinking . . .
As soon as I started looking at the good, praying, and asking God
to help me and to deliver me from all of this, all of the really bad
stuff stopped. And I felt like God had put his hands all around me
. . . It was a real miracle and I saw it as such.''

Notes

Chapter 1   *Drug Addiction: A Women's Issue*

1. Macdonald, P.T., Estep, R. Prime Time Drug Depictions. *Contemporary Drug Problems*, Fall, 1985, pp. 419-438.

2. Johnston, L.D. et. al. *Use of Licit and Illicit Drugs by America's High School Students 1975-1984.* Rockville: NIDA, 1985, p. 26.

3. *The New York Times*, February 28, 1985.

4. Prather, J.E., Fidell, L.S. Drug use and abuse among women: An overview. *International Journal of the Addictions*, 1978, *13*, pp. 863-885.

5. Burt, M., Glynn, T., Sowder, B.J. *An Investigation of the Characteristics of Drug Abusing Women.* DHEW Pub. No. (ADM) 80-917. Rockville: NIDA, 1979.

6. *Data from the Drug Abuse Warning Network (DAWN).* Series I, Number 4. Rockville: NIDA, 1985, p. 50.

7. According to figures supplied by the National Institute on Alcoholism and Alcohol Abuse (NIAAA), 1980.

8. Lester, L. The Special Needs of the Female Alcoholic. *Social Casework: The Journal of Contemporary Social Work*, October, 1982, pp. 451-456.

9. Kauffman, S.B. Marketing to Women of Tomorrow. *Market Watch*, November, 1985, p. 33.

10. Estimate provided by the New York City Health Dept, in *Los Angeles Times*, December 11, 1986, Part I, p. 1.

11. Figures provided by the State Attorney General's Bureau of Criminal Statistics. *Los Angeles Times*, March 24, 1987, I, p. 2.

12. Chambers, C.D., Hunt, L.G. Drug use patterns in pregnant women. In Rementeria, J.L., ed. *Drug Abuse in Pregnancy and the Neonate*. St. Louis: Mosley, 1977, cited in NIDA, *Treatment Services for Drug Dependent Women*, Volume 1. Rockville: NIDA, 1981, p. 28.

13. Sandmaier, M. *The Invisible Alcoholic.* New York: McGraw-Hill Book Company, 1980.

14. Quoted in Morgan, H.W. *Drugs in America: A Social History, 1800-1900*. Syracuse: Syracuse University Press, 1981.

15. Terry, C., and Pellen, M. *The Opium Problem*. Bureau of Social Hygiene. Reprinted 1970, Patterson Smith, Montclair, N.J.

16. Hughes, R., Brewing, R., *The Tranquilizing of America*. New York: Harcourt Brace Jovanovich, 1979, p. 63.

17. Cooperstock, R. Sex differences in the use of mood-modifying drugs: an explanatory model. *Journal of Health and Social Behavior*, 1971, *12*, pp. 238-244; Badiet, P. Women and legal drugs: a review. In MacLennan, A. ed. *Women: Their Use of Alcohol and Other Legal Drugs*. Toronto: Addiction Research Foundation, 1976.

18. Hughes, R., Brewin, R., 1979, p. 62.

19. Mendelsohn, R.S. *Male Practice*. Chicago: Contemporary Books, 1982, p. 60.

20. Bell, D.A. Dependence on Psychotropic Drugs and Analgesics. In Kalant, O.J., ed. *Alcohol and Drug Problems in Women*. New York: Plenum Press, 1980.

21. Broverman, I.K., Broverman, D.M., Clarkson, F.E., Rosenbranz, P.S., Bogel, S.R. Sex role stereotypes and clinical judgements of mental health. *Journal of Consulting and Clinical Psychology*, 1970, *34*, pp. 1-7.

22. Stafford, R.A., Petway, Judy M. Stigmatization of Men and Women Problem Drinkers and Their Spouses: Differential Perception and Leveling of Sex Differences. *Journal of Studies on Alcohol*, 1977, *38*, 11.

23. Belfer, M., Shader, R.I., Caroll, M., Harmatz, J.S. Alcoholism in Women. *Archives of General Psychiatry*, 1971, *25*, pp. 540-544.

24. Mendelsohn, R.S., 1982, p. 60.

Chapter 2   *Alcohol: Jill's Story*

1. Brody, J. New York Times News Service, November 17, 1985.

2. Statistics supplied by NIAAA, reported in *Time*, March 7, 1986.

3. Smith, A.R. Alcoholism and Gender: Patterns of Diagnosis and Response. *The Journal of Drug Abuse Issues*, 1986, *16* (3).

4. Kauffman, S.B. Marketing to Women of Tomorrow. *Market Watch*, November, 1985.

5. Youcha, G.A. *Women and Alcohol: A Dangerous Pleasure*. New York: Crown Publishers Inc., rev. 1986.

6. New York State Society for the Promotion of Temperance, *Annual Report,* 1832, Albany, N.Y.

7. Gough, J.B. *Autobiography and Personal Reflections*. San Francisco: Francis Dewing, 1870.

8. Smith, A.R., 1986.

9. Figures cited by Senator Paula Hawkins. See Kirkpatrick, J. *Goodbye Hangovers, Hello Life*. New York: Atheneum, 1986, p. xiv.

10. Smith, A.R., 1986.

11. Corrigan, E.M. *Alcoholic Women in Treatment*. New York: Oxford University Press, 1980.

12. Blume, S.B. Women and Alcohol. In Bratter, T.E., Forrest, G. G. eds., *Alcoholism and Substance Abuse*. New York: The Free Press, 1985.

13. Armor, D.J., Polich, J.M., and Stambul, H.B. *Alcoholism and Treatment*. New York: John Wiley & Sons, 1978; Blume, S. as quoted in *Los Angeles Times*, September 21, 1986.

14. Schmidt, W. and De Lint, J. Mortality experiences of male and female alcoholic patients. *Quarterly Journal of Studies on Alcohol*, 1969, *30*, 112-118.

15. Based on autopsies performed by Dr. Paul D. Saville. See Youcha, G.A., 1986, p. 121.

16. Schatzkin, A. et. al., Alcohol consumption and breast cancer in the epidemiologic follow-up study of the first national health and nutrition examination survey. *The New England Journal of Medicine*, May 7, 1987, 316 (19), 1169-1173.

17. Willett, W.C. et. al., Moderate alcohol consumption and the risk of breast cancer. *The New England Journal of Medicine*, May 7, 1987, 316 (19), 1174-1180.

18. Adelstein, A., White, G. Alcoholism and mortality. *Population Trends*, 1976, *6*, 7-13, cited in Willet, W.C. et. al., 1987.

19. Beckman, L. Self-esteem of woman alcoholics. *Journal of Studies on Alcohol*, 1978, *39*, 491-498.

20. Van Gelder, L. Dependencies of Independent Women. *Ms.*, February, 1987, p. 42.

21. Corrigan, E.M., 1980.

22. Blume, S.B., 1985.

23. Research Triangle Institute, *Economic Costs to Society of Alcohol and Drug Abuse and Mental Illness*. 1980, p. B-3.

24. Mills, J.L., Graubard, B.I. Is Moderate Drinking During Pregnancy Associated With an Increased Risk for Malformations? *Pediatrics*, 1987, *60* (3), pp. 309-314.

25. In a study by the American Academy of Pediatrics, reported in *New Age*, August, 1985.

26. Segal R., and Sisson, B.V. Medical Complications Associated with Alcohol Use and the Assessment of Risk of Physical Damage. In Bratter, T.E., Forrest, G.G., 1985.

27. Helzer, J.E., et. al. The Extent of Long-Term Drinking Among Alcoholics Discharged from Medical and Psychiatric Treatment Facilities. *The New England Journal of Medicine*, 1985, *312* (26), pp. 1678-1682.

28. Youcha, G.A., 1986, p. 176.

Chapter 3   *Valium: Melanie's Story*

1. Based on figures provided in *Data from the Drug Abuse Warning Network*. Rockville: NIDA, 1985, p. 26.

2. Figures supplied to the authors by DAWN.

3. Hughes, R., Brewin, R. *The Tranquilizing of America*. New York: Harcourt Brace Jovanovich, 1979, p. 66.

4. Rosenblatt, S., Dodson, R. *Beyond Valium*. New York: Putnam, 1981, p. 46.

5. Jones-Witters, P., Witters, W. *Drugs and Society*. Monterey: Wadsworth Health Sciences, 1983, p. 179.

6. *National Prescription Audit*, Ambler: IMS America, 1980, cited in Bargmann, E., Wolfe, S.M., Levin, J. *Stopping Valium*. Washington: Public Citizen Health Research Group, 1982.

7. Jones-Witters, P., Witters, W., 1983, p. 180.

8. Mendelsohn, R.S. *Male Practice*. Chicago: Contemporary Books, Inc., 1982, p. 65.

9. Rosenblatt, S., Dodson, R., 1981, p. 54.

10. Jones-Witters, P., Witters, W., 1983, p. 179.

11. Rosenblatt, S., Dodson, R., 1981, p. 44.

12. Mendelsohn, R.S., *Confessions of a Medical Heretic*. Chicago: Contemporary Books, Inc., p. 82.

13. Hughes, R., Brewin, R. 1979, p. 15-17.

14. Maletzky, B.M., Klotter, J. Addiction to diazapam, *Int. Journal of the Addictions.* 1976, *11*, 95-115.

15. Maletzky, B.M., Klotter, J., 1976.

16. *1980 Data from the Client Oriented Data Acquisition Process.* Rockville: NIDA, 1981.

17. Bargmann, E. et. al., 1982, p. 20.

18. Maletzky, B.M., Klotter, J., 1976.

19. Bargmann, E., et. al., 1982.

20. *Los Angeles Times*, Sept. 4, 1985.

21. Royce, J.E. *Alcohol Problems and Alcoholism.* New York: The Free Press, 1981.

Chapter 4   *Barbiturates and Antidepressants: Laura's Story*

1. Hambourger, W.E. A Study of the Promiscuous Use of the Barbiturates. *Journal of the American Medical Association*, April 8, 1937.

2. Cohen, S. in *Hearings Before the Subcommittee to Investigate Juvenile Delinquency of the Committee on the Judiciary*, September 17, 1969. Washington, D.C.: U.S. Government Printing Office, 1969, p. 293.

3. Jones-Witters, P., Witters, W. *Drugs and Society.* Monterey: Wadsworth Health Sciences: 1983, p. 175.

4. Matuschka, P.R. The Psychopharmacology of Addiction, in Bratter, T.E., Forrest, G.G. eds., *Alcoholism and Substance Abuse.* New York: The Free Press, 1985, p. 57.

5. Bell, D.S. Dependence on Psychotropic Drugs and Analgesics. In Kalant, O.J. ed., *Alcohol and Drug Problems in Women.* New York: Plenum Press, 1980, p. 455.

6. A study by the National Institute on Drug Abuse, 1982, cited in Kasindorf, J. Innocent Addicts: Women Hooked on Prescription Drugs. *Women's Day*, July 10, 1984, p. 62.

7. Based on figures supplied in *Data from the Drug Abuse Warning Network*, Series i, Number 4. Rockville: NIDA, 1985, p. 59.

8. Jones-Witters, P., Witters, W., 1983, p. 175.

9. Jones-Witters, P., Witters, W., 1983, p. 177.

10. Jones-Witters, P., Witters, W., 1983, p. 44.

11. Brecher, E.M. ed, *Licit & Illicit Drugs*. Boston: Little, Brown and Company, 1972, p. 249.

12. Jones-Witters, P., Witters, W., 1983, p. 175.

13. Kaufman, J.F., Shaffer, H., Burglass, M.E. The Biologic Basics: Drugs and Their Effects. In Bratter, T.E., Forrest, G.G., eds. *Alcoholism and Substance Abuse*. New York: The Free Press, 1985, pp. 117-118.

14. Wilford, B.B. *Drug Abuse*. Chicago: American Medical Association, 1981, p. 34.

15. Kaufman, J.F., Shaffer, H., Burglass, M.E., 1985, p. 118.

16. Brecher, E.M., 1972, p. 256.

17. Wilford, B.B., 1981, p. 34.

18. *Drug Dependence in Pregnancy: Clinical Management of Mother and Child*. Rockville: NIDA, 1979, pp. 22-23.

19. Brecher, E.M., 1972, p. 251.

20. *Data from the Drug Abuse Warning Network*. Series I, Number 4. Rockville: NIDA, 1985, p. 59.

21. Stern, B. *The Little Black Pill Book*. New York: Bantam, 1983, p. 252.

22. N.Y. Times News Service, May 14, 1986.

23. Hughes, R., Brewin, R. *The Tranquilizing of America*. New York: Harcourt Brace Jovanovich, 1979, p. 164.

24. Jones-Witters, P., Witters, W., 1983, p. 322.

25. Jones-Witters, P., Witters, W., 1983, p. 323.

26. Matuschka, P.R., 1985, p. 57.

Chapter 5   *Diet Pills: Diana's Story*

1. Orbach, Susie. *Fat Is a Feminist Issue*. New York: Berkley Books, 1982, p. 28.

2. Kaufman, J. et. al. *Over the Counter Pills That Don't Work*. New York: Pantheon Books, 1983, p. 71.

3. Johnston, L.D. et. al. *Use of Licit and Illicit Drugs By America's High School Students 1975-1984*. Rockville: National Institute on Drug Abuse, 1985, p. 135.

4. Spotts, J.V. and Spotts, C.A., eds. *Use and Abuse of Amphetamines and Its Substitutes*, Washington, D.C.: National Institute on Drug Abuse, 1980, p. 10.

5. Jones-Witters, P., Witters, W. *Drugs and Society*. Monterey: Wadsworth Health Services, 1983, p. 134.

6. Brecher, E.M. *Licit and Illicit Drugs*. Boston: Little, Brown and Company, 1972, p. 387.

7. Jones-Witters, P. and Witters, W., 1983, p. 134.

8. Brecher, E.M., 1972, p. 484.

9. Jones-Witters, P., Witters, W., 1983, p. 138.

10. Jones-Witters, P., Witters, W., 1983, p. 135.

11. Hughes, R. and Brewin, R. *The Tranquilizing of America*. New York: Harcourt Brace Jovanovich, 1979, p. 234.

12. Mendelsohn, R.S. *Male Practice*. Chicago: Contemporary Books, Inc., 1982, p. 60.

13. Wilford, B.B., *Drug Abuse*. Chicago: American Medical Association, 1981, p. 41.

14. Johnston, L.D., et. al., 1985, p. 9.

15. Kaufman, J., et. al., 1983, p. 81.

16. Kaufman, J., et. al., 1983, p. 81.

17. *Data from the Drug Abuse Warning Network*. Annual Data 1984, Series I, Number 4. Rockville: National Institute on Drug Abuse, 1985, p. 26.

18. Chilnick, L.D., ed. *The Little Black Pill Book*. New York: Bantam Books, 1983, p. 113; Brecher, E.M., 1972, p. 278; Bennet, G., Vourakis, C. and Woolf, D.S., eds. *Substance Abuse*. New York: John Wiley & Sons, 1983, p. 105.

19. Jones-Witters, P., Witters, W., 1983, p. 138.

20. Jones-Witters, P., Witters, W., 1983, p. 141.

21. Bennet, G., et. al., 1983, p. 60.

22. Jones-Witters, P., Witters, W., 1983, p. 139.

23. Wilford, B.B., 1981, p. 159.

24. Jones-Witters, P., Witters, W., 1983, p. 140.

25. Bennet, G., et. al., 1983, p. 60.

26. Jones-Witters, P., Witters, W., 1983, p. 140.

27. Cohen, S. et. al., eds. *Frequently Prescribed and Abused Drugs*. New York: The Hayworth Press, 1982, p. 36.

28. Chambers, C.D. and Griffey, M.S. Use of legal substances within the general population: the sex and age variables. *Addictive Diseases*, 1975, *2*, 7-9.

29. Chilnick, L.D., 1983, p. 130; Bennet, G. et. al., 1983, p. 60.

30. Booz-Allen and Hamilton, *Final Report on the Needs of and Resources for Children of Alcoholic Parents*. Rockville: NIAAA, 1974.

31. Cork, R.M., *The Forgotten Children: A Study of Children with Alcoholic Parents*. Toronto: Addiction Research Foundation, 1969.

32. Black, C., Brown, S. Kids of Alcoholics. *Newsweek*, May, 1979.

33. Black, C., Bucky, F.S., Wilder-Padilla, S. The Interpersonal and Emotional Consequences of Being an Adult Child of an Alcoholic. *International Journal of the Addictions*, 1986, *21* (2), pp. 213-231.

34. Pickens, R.W. *Children of Alcoholics*. Center City: Hazelden, 1984, p. 4.

35. Black, C. *It Will Never Happen to Me*. Denver: M.A.C., 1982, p. 141.

36. Black, C., 1982, p. 136.

37. Nici, J. Wives of Alcoholics as Repeaters. *Journal of Studies on Alcohol*, 1979, *40* (7), pp. 677-682.

38. Maria, R. Current Survey of 150 Cases. In Roy, M., ed., *Battered Women*. New York: Van Nostrand Renhold, 1977.

39. Middleton-Moz, J., Dwinell, L. *After the Tears*. Pompano Beach: Health Communications, 1986.

40. Beletsis, S., Brown, S. A Developmental Framework for Understanding the Adult Children of Alcoholics. *Journal of Addictions and Health*, 1981, *2*, pp. 187-203.

41. Cork, R.M., 1969.

42. Braun, D.K. Therapeutic Work With Children of Alcoholics. A presentation to the California Women's Conference on Alcohol and Drug Dependencies, San Diego, September 26, 1987.

43. Middleton-Moz, J., Dwinell, L., 1986.

44. *Changes*. Available from The U.S. Journal, Inc, 1721 Blount Rd., Suite #1, Pompano Beach, Florida, 33069.

Chapter 6 *Painkillers: Tricia's Story*

1. Hughes, R., Brewin, R. *The Tranquilizing of America*. New York: Harcourt Brace Jovanovich, 1979, p. 256.

2. Jones-Witters, P., Witters, W. *Drugs and Society*. Monterey: Wadsworth Health Sciences, 1983, p. 249.

3. *Drug Utilization in Office Based Practice*. Hyattsville: U.S. Department of Health and Human Services, 1982, p. 32.

4. Mendelsohn, R.S. *Male Practice*. Chicago: Contemporary Books, Inc., 1982, p. 166.

5. Mendelsohn, R.S., 1982, p. 169.

6. *National Survey on Drug Abuse: Main Findings, 1979*. Rockville: National Institute on Drug Abuse, 1980.

7. Hughes, R., Brewin, R., 1979, p. 110.

8. Brecher, E.M. *Licit & Illicit Drugs*. Boston: Little, Brown and Company, 1972, p. 11.

9. Jones-Witters, P., Witters, W., 1983, p. 235; Brecher, E.M., 1972, p. 9.

10. Jones-Witters, P., Witters, W., 1983, p. 243.

11. *Data from the Drug Abuse Warning Network*. Rockville: National Institute on Drug Abuse, 1985, Series 1, Number 4, p. 26.

12. *Data from the Drug Abuse Warning Network*. 1985, p. 52.

13. Cicero, T.J., Sex Differences in the Effects of Alcohol and Other Psychoactive Drugs on Endocrine Function. In Kalant, O.J., ed., *Alcohol and Drug Problems in Women*. New York: Plenum Press, 1980, p. 556.

14. Jones-Witters, P., Witters, W., 1983, p. 242.

15. *Data from the Drug Abuse Warning Network*. 1985, p. 52.

16. Jones-Witters, P., Witters, W., 1983, p. 244.

17. *Data from the Drug Abuse Warning Network*. 1983, p. 26, p. 52.

18. Wilford, B.B. *Drug Abuse*. Chicago: American Medical Association, 1981, p. 29.

19. Wilford, B.B., 1981, p. 151.

20. Kaufman, J.F., Shaffer, H., Burglass, M.E., The Biological Basics: Drugs and Their Effects. In Bratter, T.E., Forrest, G.G., eds., *Alcoholism and Substance Abuse*, New York: The Free Press, 1985, p. 111.

21. Beck, M., Buckley, J., Nurses With Bad Habits. *Newsweek*, August 22, 1983, p. 54.

22. Levine, D.G., Preston, P.A., Lipscomb, S.G., A historical approach to understanding drug abuse among nurses. *The American Journal of Psychiatry*, 1974, *131* (9), pp. 1036-1037.

Chapter 7   *Marijuana: Amber's Story*

1. *National Household Survey on Drug Abuse: Population Estimates 1985*. Rockville: NIDA, 1987, p. 10.

2. *Facts on File*, New York: Facts on File, Inc., 1984, p. 948.

3. *Facts on File*, 1984, p. 948.

4. Ferrence, R.G., Whitehead, P.C., Sex Differences in Psychoactive Drug Use. In Kalant, O.J., ed., *Alcohol and Drug Problems in Women*, New York: Plenum Press, 1980, p. 160.

5. *National Household Survey on Drug Abuse: Population Estimates 1985*, 1987.

6. Miller, J.D. et al., *National Survey on Drug Abuse: Main Findings 1982*. Rockville: NIDA, 1983a, p. 39.

7. Miller, J.D. et al., *Highlights from The National Survey on Drug Abuse: 1982*. Rockville: NIDA, 1983b, p. 25.

8. Miller, J.D. et al., 1983b, p. 16.

9. *Los Angeles Times*, September 25, 1986, Part I, p. 22.

10. Jones-Witters, P., Witters, W., *Drugs and Society*, Monterey: Wadsworth Health Sciences, 1983, p. 124.

11. Moran, C. Depersonalization and agoraphobia associated with marijuana use. *British Journal of Medical Psychology*, June, 1986, Vol. 59, Part 2, pp. 187-196.

12. *Los Angeles Times*, December 28, 1987.

13. Finnegan, L.P., Fehr, K.O., The Effects of Opiates, Sedative-hypnotics, Amphetamines, Cannabis, and Other Psychoactive Drugs on the Fetus and Newborn. In Kalant, O.J., ed., *Alcohol and Drug Problems in Women*, New York: Plenum, 1980, p. 691.

Chapter 8   *Cocaine: Nanci's Story*

1. *The New York Times*, February 28, 1985.

2. From a study in the *Journal of the American Medical Association*, reported in *Los Angeles Times*, July 5, 1985.

3. *Los Angeles Times*, July 5, 1985.

4. *Data from the Drug Abuse Warning Network*. Series I, Number 4, Rockville: NIDA, 1985, p. 26, p. 52.

5. *Use of Licit and Illict Drugs by America's High School Students 1975-1984*. Rockville: NIDA, 1985, pp. 11, 25.

6. *Science Digest*, April, 1985, p. 20.

7. *The New York Times*, February 18, 1985.

8. *The New York Times*, February 18, 1985.

9. *The New York Times*, February 18, 1985.

10. *The New York Times*, February 18, 1985.

11. Orth, M. Women & Cocaine. *Vogue*, November, 1984, p. 240.

12. *Los Angeles Times*, December 4, 1986, Part I, p. 4.

13. *Los Angeles Times*, September 25, 1986, Part I, p. 22.

14. Holbrok, J.M. CNS Stimulants. In Bennet, G., Vourakis, C., Woolf, D.S., eds. *Substance Abuse*. New York: John Wiley & Sons, 1983, p. 63.

15. Study in *New England Journal of Medicine*, reported in *Discover*, December, 1985, p. 9.

16. *Los Angeles Times*, December 11, 1986, Part I, p. 1.

17. *Los Angeles Times*, December 5, 1985, Part I, p. 37.

18. Gold, M.S., *800-Cocaine*. New York: Bantam, 1984, p. 11.

19. Leishman, K. Heterosexuals and AIDS. *The Atlantic Monthly*, February, 1987, p. 55.

Chapter 9   *Crack: Lindy's Story*

1. *Los Angeles Times*, September 25, 1986.

2. *Los Angeles Times*, July 31, 1986, Part I, p. 1.

3. Lamar J.V., Jr. Crack. *Time*, June 2, 1986, p. 16-18.

4. *Los Angeles Times*, September 25, 1986.

5. *Los Angeles Times*, February 14, 1987.

6. Kerr, P. Crack Addiction: The Tragic Impact on Women and Children in New York. *The New York Times*, February 9, 1987.

7. Kerr, P., 1987.

8. Black, L., Burke, D. Crack's Deadly Cycle. *Maclean's*, September 29, 1986, pp. 44-45.

9. Cohen, S. The Implications of Crack. *Drug Abuse & Alcoholism Newsletter*, July 1986.

10. Lieber, J. Coping With Cocaine. *The Atlantic Monthly*, January, 1986, pp. 39-48.

11. Black, L., Burke, D., 1986, pp. 44-45.

12. *Facts on File*, August 15, 1986, p. 601.

13. *The New York Times*, November 20, 1986, p. 16.

14. Starr, D. Cocaine antidote. *Omni*, November, 1986, p. 50.

15. Gold, M.S., Dackis, C.A., Pottash, A.L.C., Extein, I., Washton, A. Cocaine Update: From Bench to Bedside. *Advances in Alcohol and Substance Abuse*, 1986, *5* (1/2), pp. 35-61.

16. Seligman, J., McKillop, P., Greenberg, N.F., Burgower, B. Crack: The Road Back. *Newsweek*, June 30, 1986, pp. 52-53.

Chapter 10   *Crystal: Sissy's Story*

1. Smith, R.C. The Marketplace of Speed: Violence and Compulsive Methamphetamine Abuse. Unpublished, 1969, cited in Spotts, J.V. and Spotts, C.A. *Use and Abuse of Amphetamine and its Substitutes*. Rockville: NIDA, 1980, p. 11.

2. Smith, R.C., 1969.

3. Figure supplied by a DEA official, in Meyer, J.S. 'Finest city' is now crystal meth capital. *The San Diego Union*, November 18, 1985.

4. Figures supplied by California State Attorney General, *The San Diego Union*, April 22, 1987.

5. Meyer, J.S., 1985.

6. *Chemical Engineering News*, No. 3, 1969, p. 11.

7. Smith, R.C., 1969.

8. Smith, R.C., 1969, cited in Brecher, E.M. *Licit and Illicit Drugs.* Boston: Little, Brown and Company, 1972, p. 288.

9. *Data from the Drug Abuse Warning Network (DAWN).* Series I, Number 5. Rockville: NIDA, 1986. pp. 35, 62.

10. Hofmann, F.G. *A Handbook on Drug and Alcohol Abuse.* New York: Oxford University Press, Second Edition, 1983, p. 233.

11. Smith, R.C. Speed and Violence: Compulsive Methamphetamine Abuse and Criminality in the Haight-Ashbury District. In Zarafonetis, C.J.D. *Drug Abuse: Proceedings of the International Conference.* Philadelphia: Lea & Febiger, 1972, pp. 435-448.

12. Kramer, J.C. et. al. Amphetamine abuse: Pattern and effects of high doses taken intravenously. *Journal of the American Medical Association,* July 31, 1967, pp. 305-309.

13. Smith, R.C., 1969, in Brecher, 1972, p. 284.

14. Smith, R.C., 1972.

15. Stages 2 through 4 are discussed in Hofmann, F.G., 1983.

16. Kramer, J.C. et. al., 1967.

17. Kramer, J.C. et. al., 1967.

18. Jones-Witters, P., Witters, W. *Drugs and Society.* Monterey: Wadsworth Health Sciences, 1983, p. 139.

19. Kramer, J.C. Introduction to Amphetamine Abuse. *Journal of Psychedelic Drugs,* 2 (2), 1969.

20. Frykman, J.H. The Operation of a Community-Based Treatment Program. In Zarafonetis, C.J.D., ed. *Drug Abuse: Proceedings of the International Conference.* Philadelphia: Lea & Febiger, 1972, pp. 527-543.

21. Kramer, J.C. Some Observations on and a Review of the Effects of High-Dose Use of Amphetamines. In Zarafonetis, C.J.D., ed. *Drug Abuse: Proceedings of the International Conference.* Philadelphia: Lea & Febiger, 1972, pp. 253-261.

Chapter 11 *Heroin: Kit's Story*

1. National Institute on Drug Abuse, *Epidemiology of Heroin: 1964-1984.* Rockville: NIDA, 1985, p. 1.

2. Estimates by the U.S. Drug Enforcement Administration, in *Newsweek,* April 13, 1987, p. 63.

3. *Facts on File*. New York: Facts on File, Inc, 1984, p. 948.

4. Martin, C.A., Martin, W.R. Opiate Dependence in Women. In Kalant, O.J. ed. *Alcohol and Drug Problems in Women*, New York: Plenum Press, 1980, p. 465.

5. Based on an estimate that only ten percent of heroin users are true addicts, see Jones-Witters, P., Witters, W. *Drugs and Society*. Monterey: Wadsworth Health Sciences, 1983, p. 241.

6. Prather, J.E., Fidell, L.S. Drug use and abuse among women: An overview. *International Journal of the Addictions*, 1978, *13*, p. 863-885.

7. *Data from the Drug Abuse Warning Network*. Series I, Numbers 3 & 4, Rockville: NIDA, 1984, 1985, p. 47 (1984), p. 52 (1985).

8. Martin, C.A., Martin, W.R., 1980, p. 468.

9. Martin, C.A., Martin, W.R., 1980, p. 469.

10. Cuskey, W.R., Wathey, R.B. *Female Addiction*. Lexington: Lexington Books, 1982, p. 3.

11. New York City Health Department estimate, *Los Angeles Times*, December 11, 1986, Part I, p. 1.

12. *Data from the Drug Abuse Warning Network*. Series I, Number 4, Rockville: NIDA, 1985, p. 71.

13. *Report of the President's Commission on Mental Health*. 1978.

14. Terry, C., Pellens, M. The extent of chronic opiate abuse in the United States prior to 1921. In Ball. J., Chambers, C.D., eds. *The Epidemiology of Opiate Addiction in the United States*. Springfield: Charles C. Thomas, 1970.

15. NIDA, *Epidemiology of Heroin: 1964-1984*, p. 2.

16. NIDA, *Epidemiology of Heroin: 1964-1984*, p. 39.

17. Guinan, M. E., Hardy, A. Epidemiology of AIDS in Women in the United States. *Journal of the American Medical Association, 257* (15) April 17, 1987, p. 2039-2042.

18. *Time*, August 12, 1985, p. 42.

19. *Los Angeles Times*, March 27, 1987, I, p. 17.

20. *Facts on File*, 1984, p. 738.

21. Reed, B.G. Intervention Strategies for Drug Dependent Women: An Introduction. In Beschner, G.M., Reed, B.G., Mondanaro, J., eds., *Treatment Services for Drug Dependent Women*, Rockville: NIDA, 1981, pp. 8, 14.

22. In San Diego, for example, chemically dependent addicts wait up to six months. *Los Angeles Times*, December 12, 1986, Part II, p. 1.

Chapter 12 *The Pattern of Experience*

1. Reed, B.G. Intervention Strategies for Drug Dependent Women: An Introduction. In Beschner, G.M., Reed, B.G., Mondanaro, J., eds. *Treatment Services for Drug Dependent Women*, Vol. I. Rockville: National Institute on Drug Abuse, 1982, pp. 1-24.

2. Davidson, V., Bemko, J. International Review of Women and Drug Abuse (1968-1975). *Journal of American Medical Women's Association*, 1978, *33*(12), pp. 507-515.

3. Beckman, L.J. The Psychosocial Characteristics of Alcoholic Women. *Drug Abuse and Alcoholism Review*, 1978, *1* (5/6), pp. 1-12.

4. Gomberg, E.S. Drinking Patterns of Women Alcoholics, in Burtle, V., ed. *Women Who Drink*. Springfield: Charles C. Thomas, 1979, pp. 26-48.

5. Levy. A.J., Doyle, K.M. Attitudes towards women in a drug abuse treatment program. *Journal of Drug Issues*, 1974, *4*, pp. 428-435.

6. Schultz, A.M. Radical feminism: A treatment modality for addicted women. In Senay, E., Shorty, V., Alkesne, H., eds. *Developments in the Field of Drug Abuse*. Cambridge: Schenkman, 1975, cited in Beschner, G.M., Reed, B.G., Mondanaro, J., eds. *Treatment Services for Drug Dependent Women*, Vol. I. Rockville: National Institute on Drug Abuse, 1982, p. 26.

7. Cuskey, W.R., Wathey, R.B. *Female Addiction*. Lexington: Lexington Books, 1982, p. 19.

8. Marsh, J.C. Public Issues and Private Problems: Women and Drug Use. *Journal of Social Issues*, 1982, *38* (2), pp. 153-165.

9. Chambers, C.D., Inciardi, J.A., Seigal, H.A. *Chemical Coping: A report on legal drug use in the United States*. New York: Spectrum Publications, 1975, in Marsh, J.C., 1982, p. 55.

10. Authors' survey.

11. Authors' survey.

12. Schaef, A.W. *Women's Reality*. San Francisco: Harper & Row, 1981, p. 27.

13. Kohn, A. Shattered Innocence, *Psychology Today*, February, 1987, p, 54.

14. Stoenner, H., *Child Abuse Seen Growing in the United States*. Denver: American Humane Association, 1972.

15. Trotter, R.J. Fathers and Daughters: The broken bond. *Psychology Today*, March 1985, p. 10.

16. Kohn, A., 1987.

17. Benward, J., Densen-Gerber, J. *Incest as a Causative Factor in Anti-Social Behavior: An Exploratory Study*. New York: Odyssey Institute, 1975.

18. Cited by Covington, S.S. Alcohol and Family Violence. Presented at the 29th International Institute on the Prevention and Treatment of Alcoholism, Zagreb, Yugoslavia, 1983. Unpub.

19. Herman, J.L., Hirschman, L. *Father-Daughter Incest*. Cambridge: Harvard University Press, 1981, p. 93.

20. See Bass, E., Thornton, L., *I Never Told Anyone*, New York: Harper & Row, 1983, pp. 25-26.

21. Lindberg F.H., Distad, L.J. Post-Traumatic Stress Disorders in Women Who Experienced Childhood Incest. *Child Abuse & Neglect*, 1985, *9*, pp. 329-334.

22. Cuskey, W.R., Wathey, R.B., 1982, p. 136.

23. Miller, J., Moeller, D., Kaufman, A., Recidivism among sex assault victims. *American Journal of Psychiatry*, 1978, *135*, pp. 1103-1104.

24. Herman, J.L., Hirschman, L., 1981, p. 99.

25. Herman, J.L., Hirschman, L., 1981, p. 101.

26. Goodwin, J., McCarty, T., DiVasto, P., Prior incest in abusive mothers. *Child Abuse & Neglect*, 1981, *5*, pp. 1-9.

27. Herman, J.L., Hirschman, L., 1981, p. 103.

28. For a state-by-state listing of programs offering help to survivors of incest, see Ellen Bass and Louise Thornton's *I Never Told Anyone*, cited above.

29. Reed, B.G., 1982.

30. Sanford, L.T., Donovan, M.E. *Women & Self-Esteem*. New York: Penguin Books, 1985, p. 5.

31. Covington, S.S., 1983, p. 66.

32. Figures cited by Watts, D.L., Courtois, C.A. Trends in the Treatment of Men Who Commit Violence against Women. *The Personnel and Guidance Journal*, December, 1981, pp. 245-249.

33. Steinmetz, S.K., cited in Watts & Courtois, 1981.

34. Longley, R., Levy, C.L. *Wife Beating*. New York: E.P. Dutton, 1977, p. 72.

35. Scott, P.D. Battered Wives. *British Journal of Psychiatry*, 1974, *125*, pp. 433-441.

36. Carpenter, E., 1986.

37. Figure cited by Walker, L.E. *The Battered Woman Syndrome*. New York: Springer, 1984, p. 47.

38. Hanneke, C.R., Shields, N.A. Marital Rape: Implications For the Helping Professions. *Social Casework: The Journal of Contemporary Social Work*, October, 1985, pp. 451-458.

39. Finkelhor, D., Yllo, K. Rape in Marriage: A Sociological View, in Finkelhor, D., Gelles, R.J., Hotaling, G.T., Straus, M.A., eds. *The Dark Side of Families: Current Family Violence Research*. Beverly Hills: Sage Publication, 1983, pp. 119-130, cited in Hanneke and Shields.

40. Walker, L.E., 1984, p. 49.

41. Berk, R., Newton, P., *American Sociological Review, 50* (2).

42. Carpenter, E. Traumatic bonding and the battered wife. *Psychology Today*, August 14, 1986, p. 18.

43. Seligman, M.E. Depression and learned helplessness. In Friedman, R.J., Katz, N.M., eds. *The Psychology of Depression: Contemporary Theory and Research*. Washington, D.C.: Winston, 1974.

44. Smith, A.R. Alcoholism and Gender: Patterns of Diagnosis and Response. *The Journal of Drug Abuse Issues*, 1986, *16* (3), pp. 407- 420.

45. Doyle, K.M. Assertiveness Training for the Drug Dependent Woman, in Reed, B.G., Beschner, G.M., Mondanaro, J., eds., 1982, pp. 213-246.

46. Long, V.O. *Journal of Consulting and Clinical Psychology*, 1986, *54* (3).

47. Wolfe, J.L., 1979, in Burtle, V., ed. *Women Who Drink*. Springfield: Charles C. Thomas, 1979, p. 206.

48. Soler, E., Ponsor, L., Adob, J. Women in Treatment: Client Self-Report, in *Women in Treatment: Issues and Approaches*. Arlington: National Drug Abuse Center for Training and Resource Development, 1976, pp. 31-47.

49. Wolfe, J.L. A Cognitive/Behavioral Approach to Working with Women Alcoholics, in Burtle, V., ed., 1979, pp. 197-216.

50. Lee, D.L. Alcoholism Among Third World Women: Research and Treatment. In Burtle, V., 1979, p. 98.

51. Leland, J., Alcohol Use and Abuse in Ethnic Minority Women. In Wilsnack, S.C., Beckman, L.J. *Alcohol Problems in Women*. New York: Guilford Press, 1984, p. 126.

52. Gary, L.E., Gary, R.B. Treatment Needs of Black Alcoholic Women, in Brisbane, F.L., Womble, M., eds. *Treatment of Black Alcoholics*. New York: The Hayworth Press, 1985, p. 101.

53. Leland, J., 1984, p. 126.

54. Lee, D.L., 1979, p. 99.

55. Wechsler, H. Epidemiology and Male/Female Drinking. Paper presented at NIAAA Workshop on Alcoholism and Alcohol Abuse Among Women, Jekyll Island, Ga., April 2-5, 1978. Cited in Sandmaier, M., 1980.

56. Lee, D.L., 1979, p. 107.

57. Data from the Drug Abuse Warning Network (DAWN). Rockville: NIDA, 1983, p. 42.

58. Westermeyer, J. "The Drunken Indian": Myths and Realities. In Unger, S., ed. *Destruction of American Indian Families*, New York: Association on American Indian Affairs, 1977.

59. Youcha, G.A. *Women and Alcohol*. New York: Crown Publishers, 1978, pp. 19-20.

60. Alcohol and Native Americans. *Alcohol Topics: research review*. Rockville: National Clearinghouse for Alcohol Information, September, 1985.

61. National Institute on Alcohol Abuse and Alcoholism Advisory Council, "Minutes of Advisory Council Meeting," 23 May 1977, p. 2, as cited in Sandmaier, p. 147.

62. Sandmaier, M., 1980, p. 148.

63. Jones, L. Personal communication. Los Angeles Indian Lodge Detox, Los Angeles, California, March, 1977, cited in Burtle, V., 1979, p. 109.

64. Minutes of NIAAA Advisory Council Meeting, as cited in Sandmaier, M., 1980, pp. 148-149.

65. Rosenbaum, M. Sex roles among deviants: The woman addict. *International Journal of the Addictions*, 1981, *16* (5), pp 859-877.

66. Lee, D.L., 1979, p. 107.

67. Rosenbaum, M. 1981, pp. 870-874.

68. Brooks, V.R. *Minority Stress and Lesbian Women.* Lexington: Lexington Books, 1981, p. 91.

69. Saghir, M.T. Cited in Sandmaier, M. pp. 179-180.

70. Fifield, L. On My Way to Nowhere: Alienated, Isolated, and Drunk— An Analysis of Gay Alcohol Abuse and an Evaluation of Alcoholism Rehabilitation Services for the Los Angeles Gay Community. 1975. Unpublished paper. Office on Alcohol Abuse and Alcoholism, Los Angeles County Health Services.

71. Mills, B.B., Nelson, M.B. Perspectives on Treatment of Drug Dependent Lesbians, in Reed, B.G., Beschner, G.M., Mondanaro, J., eds., *Treatment Services for Drug Dependent Women*, Vol. II, Rockville: NIDA, 1982, p. 443.

72. Cuskey. W.R., Wathey, R.B., 1982, p. 19.

73. Chinlund. S. Drug addiction: Implications for illegitimacy. In *Illegitimacy: Changing Services for Changing Times.* New York: National Council on Illegitimacy, 1970; Waldorf, D. *Careers in Dope.* Englewood Cliffs: Prentice Hall, 1973. Both cited in Reed, B.G., Beschner, G.M., Mondanaro, J., eds., 1982, p. 443.

74. Cuskey, W.R., Premkumar, T., Sigel, L. Survey of opiate addiction among females in the United States between 1850 and 1970. *Public Health Reviews*, 1972, *1*, pp. 8-39.

75. Weisman, M. In a talk to the Fifth Annual Conference on Alcohol and Chemical Dependency, February 17, 1985, The Betty Ford Center, Rancho Mirage, California.

76. Hyde, J.S., Rosenberg, B.G. *Half the Human Experience: The Psychology of Women.* Washington, D.C.: Heath Company, 1980; Rosen, D.H. *Lesbianism: A Study of Female Homosexuality.* Springfield: Charles C. Thomas, 1974. Both cited in Reed, B.G., Beschner, G.M., Mondanaro, J., eds., 1982, p. 444.

77. Spence, J.T., Helmreich, R. *Masculinity and Femininity.* Austin: University of Texas Press, 1978. Cited in Reed, B.G., Beschner, G.M., Mondanaro, J., eds., 1982, p. 444.

78. In a private communication, October 4, 1987.

79. Finnegan, D.G., McNally, E.B. *Dual Identities: Counseling Chemically Dependent Gay Men and Lesbians.* Minneapolis: Hazelden, 1987, p. 38.

80. Lester, L. The Special Needs of the Female Alcoholic. *Social Casework*, 1982, *63* (8), pp. 451-456.

81. Curlee, J.A. A comparison of male and female patients at an alcoholism treatment center. *Journal of Psychology*, 1970, *74*, pp. 239-247.

82. Gomberg, E.S. Problems with alcohol and other drugs. In Gomberg, E., Franks, V., eds. *Gender and Disordered Behavior*. New York: Brunner/Mazel, 1979, in Marsh, J.C., Miller, N.A., 1985, cited below.

83. Tucker, B.M. A description and comparative analysis of the social support structure of heroin addicted women. In *Addicted Women: Family Dynamics, Self Perceptions and Support Systems*. DHEW Pub. No. (ADM) 80-762, Rockville: National Institute on Drug Abuse, 1979. Cited in Beschner, G.M., et. al. 1981, p. 33.

84. Marsh, J.C., Miller, N.A. Female Clients in Substance Abuse Treatment. *The International Journal of the Addictions*, 1985, *20* (6&7), pp. 995-1019.

85. Colten, M.E. Attitudes, experiences and self perceptions of heroin-addicted women. *Journal of Social Issues*, 1982, *38* (2), pp. 77-92 in Marsh & Miller, p. 1000.

86. Reed, B.G., 1982, p. 8.

87. Marsh, J.C., Miller, N.A., 1985.

88. Beschner, G., Thompson, P. *Women and Drug Abuse Treatment Needs and Service*. Rockville: National Institute on Drug Abuse, 1981, p. 5.

89. Harris, S. Mothers in methadone programs need day care. In Senay, E., Shorty, V., Alkesne, H., eds., 1975. Cited in Beschner, G., Thompson, P., 1981, p. 6.

90. Ryan, V.S. Differences Between Males and Females in Drug Treatment Programs. Ann Arbor: Women's Drug Research Project, University of Michigan, 1979. Cited in Beschner, G., Thompson, P., 1981, p. 5.

91. Beschner, G., Thompson, P., 1981, p. 20.

92. Levy, S.T., Doyle, K. Attitudes toward women in drug abuse treatment programs. Paper presented at the First National Drug Abuse Conference, Chicago, March, 1974, cited in Marsh, 1982.

93. Beschner, G., Thompson, P., 1981, p. 5.

94. National Institute on Drug Abuse. *Data from the Client Oriented Data Acquisition Process (CODAP)*. Series D., No. 13, Rockville: NIDA, 1979.

95. Cited in Alcoholics Anonymous, *Pass It On*. New York: Alcoholics Anonymous World Services, Inc., 1984, p. 384.

About the Authors

Emanuel Peluso was born in Brooklyn, New York. He has published several plays, was awarded an Obie Award for distinguished writing, and was the recipient of a Rockefeller Grant for playwrights. For two years he taught writing at Rutgers University. Emanuel holds a master's degree in counseling psychology, and has counseled incestuous families and crime victims, as well as recovering drug abusers. He is presently a chemical dependency counselor at an adolescent treatment program in San Diego.

Lucy Silvay Peluso was born and brought up in Manhattan, graduated from Sarah Lawrence College, and worked for twelve years as an actress in off-off- and off-Broadway productions. She is host-moderator of a cable TV talk show and is Community Outreach Coordinator for San Diego's National Council on Alcoholism. Lucy holds an M.A. in counseling psychology, counsels recovering and co-dependent people, and is the coordinator for a woman's drug and alcohol outpatient program.

Lucy and Emanuel are both marriage, family, and child counseling registered interns. Married for eighteen years, they live in San Diego with their two teen-age children.

Resources for Sound Recovery

It Must Be Five O'Clock Somewhere   Sylvia Cary
When you're in the happiness business, nothing can go
wrong, can it? That's what psychotherapist Sylvia Cary and
her psychiatrist husband thought, but eventually, just about
everything went wrong. Here's Sylvia Cary's own story of
her marriage, her headlong tumble into alcohol and drug
addiction, and her inspiring recovery. (BO3384, $8.95)

I Never Saw the Sun Rise   Joan Donlan
Illustrations by the author.
The private, as-it-happened journal of a 15-year-old girl and
her growing dependence on drugs and alcohol. Partly
written while she was heavily involved with drugs and partly
during and after treatment for drug dependency, this is a
hopeful, true story of adolescent addiction and recovery.
(B03020, $7.95)

I'm Black and I'm Sober   Chaney Allen
The autobiography of a Black woman alcoholic. Minister's
daughter Chaney Allen shares her experiences from the
soup kitchens of Selma and the tenements of Cincinnati
to recovery and a career as an alcoholism counselor.
(B03012, $7.95)

To order by credit card, please call toll-free 1-800-328-3330.
In Minnesota, call collect (612) 559-4800. Ask for our
FREE color catalog, filled with books, tapes, films and
more, all designed to help you live healthy and free.

INDEX

Abandonment, 194
Abdominal cramps, 153
Abortion, 108, 120
Abuse. *See* Child abuse; Emotional abuse;
 Family violence; Incest; Physical abuse;
 Sexual abuse; Therapist, abuse by; Verbal
 abuse
Abusive men, attracting, 45
Access to drugs. *See* Tricia's story
Acid. *See* LSD
Acupuncture in cocaine therapy, 139
Addiction
 to BZPs, 35
 and men, 183
 physical, 24, 93
 psychological, 23, 93, 152
 and women, 183-198
Adolescent use, 19, 37-38, 155-162
Adrenalin-mimic, 71
 Adjustment reaction, 75
Adult Children of Alcoholics (ACA), 57,
 74-77, 96-97, 111, 113, 116, 155
 arrest rates of, 74
 and marijuana use, 111
Aggression, 153. *See also* Sissy's story
Aging accelerated, 110
Agitation, 73. *See also* Anxiety
Agoraphobia, 45
AIDS, (Auto-Immune Deficiency
 Syndrome), 121, 163-165
Alanon, 75
Alateen, 75
Alcohol, 1-13, 15-36. *See also* Cross
 addiction
 high tolerance for, 38
 in history, 15-16
 men and, 16
 and pharmaceutical products, 18
 and women
  age of use, 15
  attitudes about, 15
  cross addiction, 18
  physical effects, 16
  pregnancy, 17
  and relationships, 21-24
  secret drinkers, 16, 19
  and Valium cure, 36
  and women, 4
Alcoholics Anonymous (AA), 4, 17-18, 29-
 31, 43, 66-67, 86, 106, 117
 misuse of, 43
Alertness, 71
Allen, Chaney, 195-196
Amends, making, 135, 147

American Medical Association, 33, 53
Amitril, 55
Amitripyline, 55
Amphetamine, 1-13, 36, 39, 43, 45, 59, 61,
 71, 113, 151-162. *See also* Crystal
 boredom repressor, 72
 history of, 71-76
 and men, 72
 Speed, history of, 151
 and women, 72
Anger, 1-2
Anger and survival, 178-179
Analgesics, narcotic, 91
Antabuse, 18, 28
Antidepressants, 53, 55
 effect of, 55
 tricyclic, 55
Anxiety, 17, 34-35, 45, 49, 53-54, 73, 92,
 100, 112
Arrest. *See* Jail; Police; Prison
Arterial damage, 153
Arthritis symptoms, 61
Asian-American women, 191
Aspirin, 57, 91
Assertiveness skills, 184, 190
Ativan, 34
Auto-Immune Deficiency Syndrome. *See*
 AIDS
Awareness, 196

Barbiturates, 6, 53-70, 153
 history of, 53
 speech slurred, 54
Battering, 56, 64, 75, 184, 188-189
Benadryl, shooting, 175
Bennies. *See* Amphetamine
Benzodiazepine (BZP), 34
Betty Ford Center, 193
Beyond Valium (Rosenblatt and Dodson),
 34
Binging, 121
Biological prejudice, 11-12
Birthing, 91. *See also* Fetal; Miscarriages
Bisexual, 165, 193
Black beauties, 126
Blackouts, 22-23, 40, 62, 65, 124
Black women
 and Crack, 138
 and heroin, 164
 and treatment, 191-192
Blaming. *See* Parents
Blood pressure
 fetal, 121
 high, 16
 low, 55